International Coding Index
for Dermatology

Compatible with the 9th Revision
of the WHO International Classification
of Disease

Compiled by

SUZANNE ALEXANDER

Consultant Dermatologist to Ilford and
Barking Hospital and Honorary Lecturer in
the Department of Medicine
Guy's Hospital, London

and

ALAN B SHRANK

Consultant Dermatologist to the
Salop Area Health Authority

Published for the
British Association of Dermatologists
by Blackwell Scientific Publications
Oxford London Edinburgh Melbourne

© 1978 British Association of Dermatologists
and published for them by
Blackwell Scientific Publications
Osney Mead, Oxford, OX2 0EL
8 John Street, London WC1N 2ES,
9 Forrest Road, Edinburgh EH1 2QH,
P.O. Box 9, North Balwyn, Victoria, Australia.

First published 1978

British Library Cataloguing in Publication Data

Alexander, Suzanne
    International coding index for dermatology.
    1. Skin — Diseases
    I. Title II. Shrank, Alan B III. British
    Association of Dermatologists
    616.5'001'2   RL39

    ISBN 0-632-00272-7

Distributed in the United States of America by
J.B. Lippincott Company, Philadelphia
and in Canada by
J.B. Lippincott Company of Canada Ltd, Toronto.

Set by Getset Ltd,
Eynsham, Oxford and
printed and bound in Great Britain at
Billing & Sons Ltd, Guildford and Worcester.

Introduction

The prime aim of any system of coding of medical diagnosis is the accurate and efficient retrieval of information. To be useful for epidemiological studies, for the planning of health services and for medical research, it must be universally acceptable and understood. It must also be simple to operate.

The ICD issued by WHO works on these assumptions, but for the convenience of dermatologists this book (1976) was designed so that coding would be easier and more complete for them. The ICD is not based entirely on etiology, and no attempt has been made to alter this in the dermatological codes. The value of the current ICD is limited because many skin diseases are not recorded, and some recognised as separate entities are grouped together in one code, thus restricting the ease of retrieval of accurate information. An important feature of the ICD is the emphasis on the site of the lesion, whereas in dermatology the emphasis is usually upon a diagnosis; consequently, in particular, the ICD coding of benign and malignant skin tumours does not permit adequate separation of entities, and this has been reviewed.

The index of dermatological diagnoses includes most of the terms used in the current ICD as well as many from recent dermatological literature. Several diagnostic terms used in the ICD have been excluded on the grounds of economy and lack of universality; these comprise lay terms of inadequate definition (e.g. rash), eponymous terms of purely local value where an internationally accepted term is preferred (e.g. N. American blastomycosis for Gilchrist's disease), and rare titles for diseases with common names (e.g. maculae ceruleae for pubic lice infestation). Where symptoms or signs form only part of a diagnosis they are omitted. In this way the booklet has been made compact yet inclusive, and cross reference for many diagnoses has been preserved.

The ICD uses a decimal system with the first three digits describing the category of disease, and these have not been altered in any way. Diseases of the skin and subcutaneous tissue have been allocated the numbers 680 to 709. The other numbers also describe many skin diseases which have systemic manifestations so that the whole ICD has been abstracted. Subdivision of category numbers is by fourth digits, but this is inadequate for proper dermatological definition, so that fifth and sixth digits have been used where necessary. It would prove unwieldy to allocate a different number for each disease entity so that some diseases have still been grouped under one code (e.g. different types of tylosis). The inclusion of several entities under one code does not imply a common etiology, but it is usually restricted to rare disorders, and would still permit easy retrieval. Two abbreviations used in the ICD are NOS for "not otherwise specified" and NEC for "not elsewhere classified".

This booklet is in two parts. The first part is the alphabetical list with the coding figures. The figures used are compatible with the 9th Revision of the

ICD classification due to be used from January 1st 1979, but not everyone will be able to undertake the change-over promptly. For convenience of world-wide use American style spelling has been used. The second, the numerical section, lists all the additional numbers designed for improved coding, and all are six digit figures. Where there is no fourth digit in the standard ICD classification and further subdivision is required the letter "x" — recorded as a space by the computer — is used. It is also used as a sixth digit.

Thanks are due to the British Association of Dermatologists who invited us to write this booklet and in conjunction with Brocades G.B. Ltd., I.C.I. Ltd., and E.R. Squibb Ltd., have sponsored its publication, to the staff of the Statistical Division of WHO, to Dr. A.H.T. Robb-Smith for general advice and to our spouses for their tolerance.

Alan B. Shrank
Suzanne Alexander

Diagnoses Listed in Alphabetical Order

7576	Aberrant breast
7576	Aberrant nipple
7585	Abnormality, chromosome, autosome NOS
7588	sex anomaly
7599	congenital skin and appendage NOS
9190	Abrasion — superficial injury
6929	Abscess, NOS
00670x	amebic of skin
6163	Bartholin's gland
6110	breast
01705x	cold (tuberculous)
1259	filarial
683	lymph node
9985	operative wound
566	perianal
685	pilonidal
6829	skin NEC
2790	Absence of globulin
75570x	Absence of patella
7820	Absence of sensation, cold
7820	heat
7820	pain
757337	Absence of skin, congenital
2713	Absorption defect in lactose
7007	Absorption of drug through placenta
5798	Absorption of fat, disturbance of
5798	Absorption of protein, disturbance of
1254	Acanthocheilonemiasis
216x01	Acanthoma Degos — clear cell
7012	Acanthosis nigricans, acquired
757301	benign
757301	congenital
1339	Acariasis, NOS
13302x	animal
13300x	human
13301x	Norwegian
13300x	postscabetic nodules
30020x	Acarophobia
2738	Acatalasia
7441	Accessory auricle

1

7576	Accessory breast in axilla
7550	Accessory digit
7441	Accessory ear
7576	Accessory nipple
70186x	Accessory skin tag, acquired
757338	congenital
2552	Achard Thiers syndrome
1110	Achromia parasitica
1118	Acladiosis
70615x	Acne, agminata
70612x	chloracne
70610x	cystic
70618x	drug induced due to bromide
70618x	halogen other than bromide
70617x	steroid therapy
70616x	excoriée des jeunes filles
70613x	indurata
70611x	infantum
70613x	keloid
7060	necrotica
70612x	occupational
70612x	oil
69530x	rosacea
70617x	steroid induced
70612x	tar
70614x	tropical
7060	varioliformis
70610x	vulgaris
01709x	Acnitis
70186x	Acrochordon
44380x	Acrocyanosis
68680x	Acrodermatitis atrophicans
68680x	continua
68681x	enteropathica
68680x	Hallopeau
68680x	perstans
68680x	pustula continua
9850	Acrodynia
69690x	Acroerythème pustuleux
25800x	Acrogeria
757317	Acrokeratosis verruciformis
2530	Acromegaly
24680x	Acropachy thyroid
68680x	Acropustulosis
7101	Acrosclerosis
69271x	Actinic cheilitis
69271x	Actinic dermatitis
69272x	Actinic reticuloid
0390	Actinomycosis of skin

2

0390	Actinophytosis of skin
2104	Adamantinoma
2554	Addison's disease — adrenal
2893	Adenitis, NOS
683	acute
6163	Bartholin's
0172	scrophulous (tuberculous)
17399x	Adenocarcinoma of skin, NOS
1982	metastasis to skin
17396x	sweat gland
17391x	Adenoid squamous cell carcinoma of skin
217	Adenoma, nipple
2102	salivary gland
7595	sebaceum
216x12	senile sebaceous
216x29	sweat gland, NOS
216x23	apocrine
216x22	eccrine
7856	Adenopathy lymph node, NOS
0172	tuberculous
7092	Adherent scar
7781	Adiposonecrosis neonatorum
2729	Adiposis dolorosa
2599	Adiposity of endocrine origin
2780	NOS
216x29	Adnexal tumour, NOS
216x23	apocrine hidrocystoma
216x23	nevus
17396x	sweat gland carcinoma
216x11	calcifying epithelioma of Malherbe
216x01	clear cell hidradenoma
216x21	cylindroma
216x51	dermoid cyst
17396x	eccrine gland carcinoma
216x22	nevus
216x22	poroma
216x22	spiradenoma
70620x	epidermal cyst
216x22	eruptive hidradenoma
70583x	Fox Fordyce disease
216x22	hidradenoma eruptif
216x23	papilliferum
70620x	milium
216x43	nevus sebaceus (Jadassohn)
70620x	pilar cyst
216x11	pilomatrixoma
216x12	sebaceous adenoma
216x12	epithelioma
70621x	sebocystomatosis

216x12	Adnexal tumour, senile sebaceous hyperplasia
70621x	steatocystoma multiplex
216x23	syringocystadenoma papilliferum
216x20	syringoma
216x10	trichoepithelioma
216x10	trichofolliculoma
70620x	wen
2552	Adrenogenital syndrome, acquired
2552	congenital
2790	Agammaglobulinemia
7828	Ageing skin
757406	Agenesis of hair
75751x	nail
75570x	patella
757337	skin
2880	Agranulocytosis
1360	Ainhum
0501	Alastrim
27020x	Albinism
27021x	Albinoidism
7565	Albright's disease
2791	Aldrich Wiskott syndrome
709010	Alezzandrini's syndrome
27023x	Alkaptonuria
44780x	Allergide, nodular dermal
99942x	Allergy, Arthus phenomenon
69180x	atopic eczema
7082	cold
69230x	contact, due to drug
69260x	due to plants
69240x	chemical products excluding drugs
69280x	other specified agents
69289x	NOS
69508x	drug eruption, NOS
4930	immediate type, airborne
7080	bee sting
6925	food
4930	grass pollen
99940x	serum anaphylactic reaction
99943x	Shwartzmann reaction
75712x	Alligator skin disease
75745x	Allotrichia circumscriptum
704016	Alopecia aminogenic
704010	androgenetic
704012	areata
704010	biological, female
704010	male
704013	cicatricial, NOS
70482x	folliculitis decalvans

4

704013	Alopecia, cicatricial, pseudopelade
704004	radiotherapy
75740x	congenital
704010	constitutional
704003	drug
704014	mucinosa
704011	postinflammatory
0918	syphilitic (secondary)
704011	telogen
704012	totalis
704001	traction
704002	traumatic – chemical
704000	trichotillomania
704012	universalis
00670x	Amebiasis of skin, NOS
00670x	Amebic granuloma of skin
00670x	ulcer of skin
00670x	Ameboma of skin
216x36	Amelanotic nevus
2104	Ameloblastoma
0854	American leishmaniasis
2709	Aminoacid disorder, NOS
27740x	Amyloidosis
2870	Anaphylactoid purpura
1269	Ancylostomiasis
30011x	Anesthesia, hysterical
70131x	Anetoderma
7476	Aneurysm, arteriovenous peripheral
44781x	Angiitis, NOS
44780x	allergic
4464	granulomatous
44780x	hypersensitivity of skin
44780x	leukocytoclastic
44601x	necrotising
101	Angina, Vincent's
44780x	Angiodermatitis
9951	Angioedema
2777	hereditary
228x2x	Angioendothelioma, benign
17190x	malignant
27270x	Angiokeratoma, diffusum corporis
27270x	Fabry
757313	Fordyce
757313	Mibelli
757313	scrotal
21598x	Angioleiomyoma
214x0x	Angiolipoma
228x9x	Angioma NOS
228x0x	port wine

5

44892x	Angioma, senile
70910x	serpiginosum
44810x	spider
44812x	strawberry
75960x	Angiomatosis arteriovenous
75961x	encephalocutaneous
75961x	encephalofacial
75640x	Maffucci
4480	Osler Weber Rendu
75961x	Sturge Weber
9951	Angioneurotic edema
17190x	Angiosarcoma
7050	Anhidrosis
7050	Anidrosis
757333	Anidrotic ectodermal dysplasia
1269	Ankylostomiasis
	Annular erythema — see erythema
75749x	Anomaly of hair NOS
75759	Anomaly of nail NOS
70388x	Anonychia, acquired
75751x	congenital
3071	Anorexia nervosa
0220	Anthrax, cutaneous
709008	Antimony spots
7560	Aperts syndrome
5282	Aphthous stomatitis
5282	ulcer
757337	Aplasia cutis
70583x	Apocrine acne
	tumours: *see adnexal tumours*
	Appendage tumours: *see adnexal tumours*
75980x	Arachnodactyly
2276	Argentaffinoma
709008	Argyria
2660	Ariboflavinosis
70185x	Arndt Gottron syndrome
2561	Arrhenoblastoma, benign, female
2570	male
1830	malignant, female
1869	male
709008	Arsenical pigmentation
70117x	warts
69840x	Artefact
69840x	dermatitis
4402	Arteriosclerosis of extremities
4402	Arteriosclerotic gangrene
4402	ulcer
7476	Arteriovenous aneurysm, peripheral
44780x	Arteritis, allergic

4465	Arteritis, cranial
4465	giant cell
44601x	necrotising
44600x	nodose
7142	rheumatoid
0938	syphilitic
4465	temporal
7169	Arthritis NOS
7133	deformans
0985	gonococcal
2749	gouty
7133	mutilans
27023x	ochronotic
7133	psoriatic
7111	Reiter's
7140	rheumatoid
0940	syphilitic
7135	Arthropathy, Charcot not due to syphilis
0940	due to syphilis
7133	psoriatic
9194	Arthropod bites (nonvenomous)
9895	(venomous)
9194	Arthropod stings (nonvenomous)
9895	(venomous)
69505x	Ashy dermatosis (Ramirez)
6965	Asteatosis
4930	Asthma — atopic
3348	Ataxia telangiectasia
1104	Athlete's foot due to fungus infection
69180x	Atopic eczema
75740x	Atrichia congenita
44782x	Atrophie blanche
70131x	Atrophoderma follicular
70131x	macular
70102x	Pasini et Pierini
095	syphilitic
70183x	vermiculata
70101x	Atrophy hemifacial
70131x	macular
70388x	nail acquired
75751x	congenital
70180x	senile skin
70132x	steroid
6241	vulval
22994x	Atrophoderma, follicular
709008	Aurantiasis
7444	Auricular fistula
28733x	Autoerythrocyte sensitisation
2692	Avitaminosis NOS

6948	Bacterid, pustular
60789x	Balanitis, NOS
11222x	candidal
0990	Ducrey
60783x	erosiva circinata et gangrenosa
0980	gonococcal
60789x	phagadenic
60780x	xerotica obliterans
60784x	Zoon's
607896	Balanoposthitis
216x37	Balloon cell nevus
75745x	Bamboo hair
70781x	Barcoo rot
6163	Bartholin's abscess
6163	adenitis
6162	cyst
0880	Bartonellosis
17390x	Basal cell carcinoma
17390x	epithelioma
17395x	nevus syndrome
17394x	Basisquamous cell carcinoma
216x33	Bathing trunk nevus
9598	Battered baby
9598	syndrome
01711x	Bazin's disease
99930x	BCG granuloma
75743x	Beaded hair
70382x	Beau's lines
216x31	Becker's nevus
7070	Bedsore
7883	Bedwetting
9053	Bee sting
1361	Behcet's syndrome
1040	Bejel
216x11	Benign calcifying epithelioma of Malherbe
6946	Benign mucous membrane pemphigoid
2650	Beri beri
70988x	Beryllium granuloma
135x1x	Besnier's lupus pernio
69180x	Besnier's prurigo
1203	Bilharziasis, cutaneous
7560	Birdface
	Birthmark, *see nevus*
9194	Bites, centipede
9194	chigger
9060	dog
9194	flea
9194	insect, nonvenomous
9055	venomous

9050	Bites, reptile
9062	snake, nonvenomous
9050	venomous
9051	spider
9055	venomous, NOS
5293	Black hairy tongue
70610x	Blackhead
28731x	Black heel
1161	Blastomycosis, Brazilian
1174	European
1160	North American
1161	South American
3730	Blepharitis
3743	Blepharochalasis
919	Blister, traumatic
757322	Bloch Sulzberger disease
2899	Blood dyscrasia, NOS
2869	clotting defects
2739	globulin disease, NOS
2739	deficiency
2731	monoclonal
2730	polyclonal
2732	cryoglobulin
2733	macroglobulin
	leukemia, *see Leukemia*
2384	polycythemia vera
70911x	Bloom's syndrome
216x30	Blue nevus, benign
1729	malignant
228x3x	rubber bleb nevus
7826	Blushing
135x0x	Boeck's sarcoid
680	Boil
75983x	Bonnet Dechaume Blanc syndrome
7043	Book's syndrome
2329	Borst Jadassohn epithelioma
048	Boston exanthem
70986x	Botryomycosis
5287	Bowen's disease of mouth
2335	penis
2336	scrotum
2329	skin
5287	tongue
7444	Branchial fistula
1161	Brazilian blastomycosis
0855	leishmaniasis
69443x	pemphigus
7576	Breast, aberrant
6110	abscess

174x1x	Breast, carcinoma
6100	cyst
174x0x	Paget's disease
2020	Brill Symmers disease
70388x	Brittle nails, acquired
75752x	congenital
69180x	Brocq's disease
69297x	erythrose peribuccale pigmentaire
70582x	Bromhidrosis
70618x	Bromoderma
7444	Bronchogenetic cyst
2750	Bronze diabetes
216x10	Brooke's disease
0239	Brucella dermatitis
0239	erythema
9249	Bruise
5284	Buccal cyst
4431	Buerger's disease
684	Bullous impetigo
6945	pemphigoid
7350	Bunion
7432	Buphthalmia
2002	Burkitt's lymphoma
2002	tumour
9490	Burn, NOS
9491	first degree
9492	second degree
9493	third degree
2650	Burning feet syndrome
7820	sensation
5296	tongue
9983	Burst stiches (excludes puerperal [6742] , perineal or post Caesarean burst stitches [6741])
0311	Buruli ulcer
07811x	Buschke Lowenstein condyloma
7565	Ollendorf syndrome
71080x	scleredema
709001	Café au lait spot
2782	Caffey's syndrome
1252	Calabar swelling
70930x	Calcification, dystrophic
70930x	metastatic in skin
70930x	pinnal
216x11	Calcifying epithelioma of Malherbe
70930x	Calcinosis, circumscripta
70930x	cutis
70930x	universalis

70930x	Calculus of skin
700	Callosity
700	Callus
44811x	Campbell de Morgan spot
1982	Cancer en cuirasse
5281	Cancrum oris
6165	pudendi
11222x	Candidiasis of skin, flexural and NOS
11221x	chronic mucocutaneous
1120	oral
1121	vulval
11220x	Candidal granuloma
75742x	Canities, congenital
7043	premature
44891x	Capillaritis, cutaneous
103	Carate
28734x	Carbromal eruption
680	Carbuncle
2592	Carcinoid syndrome
2592	tumor
17390x	Carcinoma basal cell
17395x	nevus syndrome
17394x	basi-squamous cell
17391x	epidermoid
2329	intra-epidermal Borst Jadassohn
174x0x	Paget, of breast
1879	Paget, of genitalia
2335	Queyrat
1982	metastatic in skin
17396x	sebaceous gland
17391x	squamous cell
17396x	sweat gland
1999	Carcinomatosis
1982	in skin, secondary
2783	Carotenemia
5993	Caruncle, urethral
0783	Cat scratch fever
9063	Cauliflower ear
5790	Celiac disease
5829	Cellulitis
70987x	eosinophilic
216x37	Cellular nevus
9059	Centipede bite
1203	Cercarial dermatitis
3804	Cerumen, impacted
70981x	Chafing of skin
0862	Chagas disease
3732	Chalazion
75680x	Chalazoderma

11

0910	Chancre, hard
0990	soft
1020	yaws
68602x	Chancriform pyoderma
0990	Chancroid
70981x	Chapping of skin
7135	Charcot's joint, not due to syphilis
0940	due to syphilis
2882	Chediak Higashi syndrome
52852x	Cheilitis, NOS
69271x	actinic
52850x	angular
1120	candidal
52851x	glandular
2652	pellagra
	Cheilosis, *see cheilitis*
70580x	Cheiropompholyx
7014	Cheloid
9839	Chemical burn (*see also Burn*)
	dermatitis (*see dermatitis 692*)
3727	Chemosis
052	Chickenpox
0854	Chiclero ulcer
1338	Chiggers
9915	Chilblain
6954	lupus erythematosus
709002	Chloasma
70612x	Chloracne
2721	Cholesterolemia NOS
38000x	Chondrodermatitis nodularis helicis
7565	Chondroectodermal dysplasia
213x1x	Chondroma
1709	Chondrosarcoma
7528	Chordee congenital
0981	gonococcal
60782x	nonvenereal
7293	Christian Weber disease
2861	Christmas disease
2276	Chromaffinoma
70582x	Chromidrosis
1172	Chromoblastomycosis
1172	Chromomycosis
1110	Chromophytosis
2881	Chronic granulomatous disease (Good)
11221x	Chronic mucocutaneous candidiasis
69295x	Chronic superficial dermatitis
709008	Chrysiasis
7092	Cicatrix
5715	Cirrhosis of liver

709005	Civatte's poikiloderma
700	Clavus
216x22	Clear cell hidradenoma
2869	Clotting defects
7815	Clubbing
5293	Coated tongue
3042	Cocainism
114	Coccidioidomycosis
114	Coccidioidosis
25801x	Cockayne syndrome, dwarfism
757320	epidermolysis bullosa
7082	Cold allergy
7782	injury, neonatal
054	sore
7082	urticaria
0099	Colitis, NOS
558	allergic
0071	giardial
014	tuberculous
556	ulcerative
7108	Collagen disease, NEC
7108	nonvascular
7109	NOS
216x41	Collagenous plaques
70932x	Colloid degeneration
70931x	milium
70610x	Comedo
757318	nevus
30010x	Compensation neurosis
9999	Complication of immunisation NOS
990	of radiotherapy
9989	of surgical procedure, NOS,
4570	postmastectomy lymphedema
9985	stitch abscess
99909x	vaccination, NOS
99900x	accidental
99901x	eczema vaccinatum
99903x	gangrenous vaccinia
99902x	generalised vaccinia
99904x	NEC
99909x	NOS
216x37	Compound nevus
75080x	Condition, Fordyce mouth
75281x	genitalia
07811x	Condyloma acuminatum
07811x	Buschke Lowenstein
913	latum
913	syphiliticum
0188x	Confluent reticulated papillomatosis

757333	Congenital ectodermal defect
27710x	erythropoietic protoporphyria
7476	phlebectasia
757337	scalp defect
3729	Conjunctivitis,
4779	with hay fever
0984	gonorrhoeal
69531x	rosaceous
0770	swimming pool (viral)
076	trachomatous
216x41	Connective tissue nevus
7565	Conradi's disease
69289x	Contact dermatitis NOS
	allergic
69230x	due to drug
69240x	other chemical product
69280x	other specified agent except plants
69260x	plant
	irritant
69231x	due to drug
69241x	other chemical product
69281x	other specified agent except plants
69261x	plant
	reaction type unspecified
69239x	due to drug
69249x	other chemical product
69289x	other specified agent except plants
69269x	plant
0512	Contagious pustular dermatitis
7286	Contracture, Dupuytren
9299	Contusion, intact skin
8799	open wound
30011x	Conversion hysteria
700	Corn
7583	Cornelia de Lange syndrome
702x0x	Cornu cutaneum
70101x	Coup de sabre
5978	Cowperitis
0510	Cowpox, acquired from cow and not from vaccination
99900x	acquired accidentally from vaccination
0792	Coxsackie virus infection NOS
1021	Crab yaws
69181x	Cradle cap
4465	Cranial arteritis
1269	Creeping eruption
2774	Crigler Najjar syndrome
555	Crohn's disease
21133x	Cronkhite Canada syndrome
7101	CRST syndrome

2732	Cryoglobulinemia
1175	Cryptococcosis
2550	Cushing's syndrome
2550	Cushingoid state due to steroid therapy
9198	Cut
70930x	Cutaneous calculus
702x0x	Cutaneous horn
0854	Cutaneous leishmaniasis, American
0852	Asian
0851	Cuban
0853	Ethiopian
0850	post-kala-azar
216x53	Cutaneous meningioma
70181x	Cutis hyperelastica, acquired
75680x	congenital
7829	marmorata
70180x	rhomboidalis nuchae
757336	verticis gyrata
7825	Cyanosis
28800x	Cyclic neutropenia
216x21	Cylindroma, benign
17396x	malignant
6162	Cyst, Bartholin
7444	branchiogenic
6100	breast
7444	bronchogenetic
5284	buccal
5228	dental
216x51	dermoid of skin
1231	cysticercus
1229	echinococcal
70620x	epidermal
1229	hydatid
70620x	implantation
70620x	inclusion
3732	Meibomian
7274	mucous of digit
70620x	pilar
685	pilonidal
70620x	sebaceous
70620x	skin
7275	synovial of digit
7444	thyroglossal
7537	urachal
1231	Cysticercosis
2770	Cystic fibrosis
2281	hygroma
0785	Cytomegalic inclusion disease

15

690	Dandruff
75680x	Danlos Ehlers syndrome
69502x	Darier erythema annulare
757311	keratosis follicularis
135x0x	Roussy sarcoid
2648	vitamin A deficiency
7442	Darwin's tubercle
7583	de Lange syndrome
44811x	Morgan spot
757339	Sanctis Cacchione
7070	Decubitus ulcer
757333	Defect, ectodermal, congenital
757337	scalp, congenital
2869	Deficiency, clotting
261	dietary NOS
2599	endocrine NOS
2790	gammaglobulin
5277	salivary secretion
2739	serum protein
4439	vascular NOS
2692	vitamin NOS
704011	Defluvium capillorum
70388x	unguium
7443	Deformity, ear, NOS
7561	Klippel Feil
70389x	nail, acquired
75759x	congenital
7576	nipple
2773	Degeneration, amyloid
70932x	colloid
44783x	Degos disease
1338	Demodex folliculorum infection
061	Dengue fever
5228	Dental cyst
5227	sinus
3049	Dependence drug
2729	Dercum's disease
69299x	Dermatitis, NOS
69271x	actinic
69840x	artefacta
690	asteatotic
69180x	atopic
70181x	atrophicans, diffuse
70131x	macular
1203	cercarial
69295x	chronic, superficial
69289x	contact, NOS
	allergic
69230x	due to drug

16

69240x	Dermatitis, contact, allergic, other chemical products
69280x	other specified agent except plants
69260x	plant
	irritant
69231x	due to drug
69241x	other chemical product
69281x	other specified agent except plants
69261x	plant
	reaction type unspecified
69239x	due to drug
69249x	other chemical product
69289x	other specified agent except plants
69269x	plant
6910	diaper
690	eczematoid
1108	epidermophytosis, NOS
69298x	exfoliative
68603x	gangrenosa infantum
6940	herpetiformis
4541	hypostatic
690	infective
69239x	medicamentosa, contact, NOS
69230x	allergic
69231x	irritant
6930	systemic (*see disease type*)
1339	mite
6910	napkin
44780x	nodularis necroticans
6921	oil
70613x	papillaris capillitii
2652	pellagrous
69533x	perioral
68680x	perstans
69271x	photodermatitis, NOS
69232x	due to drug
69242x	other specified chemical product
69262x	plant
69262x	phytophotodermatitis
70912x	pigmented purpuric
69269x	plant NOS
68680x	repens
70912x	Schamberg
1203	schistosome
690	seborrheic
69296x	senile
69291x	sensitisation
69289x	shoe
4541	stasis
4541	varicose

17

68680x	Dermatitis, vegetans
1172	verrucosa
27280x	Dermatoarthritis, lipoid
216x50	Dermatofibroma
17191x	Dermatofibrosarcoma
70830x	Dermatographia
70181x	Dermatolysis acquired
75680x	congenital
1119	Dermatomycosis NOS
7103	Dermatomyositis
11085x	Dermatophytid
1104	Dermatophytosis, of foot
1100	of hair (not favus)
11080x	ide eruption
1106	kerion
1101	of nail
1105	of skin
1109	of NOS
70181x	Dermatorrhexis, acquired
75680x	congenital
69513x	Dermatosis, acute febrile, neutrophilic
69505x	ashy (Ramirez)
2329	Bowen's of skin
70980x	papulosa nigra
709009	pigmentary NOS
69296x	senile
6941	subcorneal pustular
69513x	Sweet's
70830x	Dermographism
216x51	Dermoid cyst of skin
44382x	Dermopathy, diabetic
757330	de Sanctis Cacchione syndrome
70781x	Desert sore
1103	Dhobie itch
2750	Diabetes bronze
2750	due to hemochromatosis
250	mellitus
2507	ulcer
44382x	diabetic dermopathy
44382x	microangiopathy
25073x	xanthomatosis
7999	Diagnosis deferred
6910	Diaper dermatitis
7425	Diastematomyelia
261	Dietary deficiency NOS
7550	Digit supernumerary
685	Dimple parasacral
685	postanal
032	Diphtheria

18

0328	Diphtheritic ulcer
3801	Discharge, ear
6117	nipple
4739	postnasal
6169	vaginal NOS
69290x	Discoid eczema
6954	lupus erythematosus
70388x	Discoloration of nail
2554	Disease, Addison's
7565	Albright
2773	amyloid
01711x	Bazin
757322	Bloch Sulzberger
2329	Bowen of skin
2020	Brill Symmers
69180x	Brocq
216x10	Brooke
4431	Buerger
0783	cat scratch
5790	celiac
0862	Chagas
7293	Christian Weber
2861	Christmas
7108	collagen NEC
7109	collagen NOS
7565	Conradi
555	Crohn
2550	Cushing
69502x	Darier erythema annulare
757311	Darier keratosis follicularis
44783x	Degos
2729	Dercum
27240x	Fabry
2729	Farber
2770	fibrocystic
0570	fifth
70583x	Fordyce Fox
0578	fourth
70583x	Fox Fordyce
0991	Frei
2724	Gaucher
2881	Good
2881	granulomatous (Good)
757321	Hailey Hailey
0743	hand, foot and mouth
2778	Hand, Schuller Christian
0309	Hansen NOS
2700	Hartnup
2019	Hodgkin

19

27760x	Disease, Hurler
70115x	Kyrle
2025	Letterer Siwe
70912x	Majocchi
757331	mast cell
7570	Milroy
75715x	Mljet
2724	Niemann Pick
4480	Osler Weber Rendu
174x0x	Paget of breast
1879	of genitalia
174x0x	of nipple
1879	of scrotum
60782x	Peyronie
9850	pink
7595	Pringle
4430	Raynaud
2377	Recklinghausen (nerves)
0993	Reiter
757332	Rothmund Thomson
70912x	Schamberg
2022	Sézary
0578	sixth
6941	Sneddon Wilkinson
7143	Still
757332	Thomson
7999	undiagnosed
1321	vagabond
	vascular
4409	arteriosclerotic
4431	obliterative
2377	von Recklinghausen (nerves)
7293	Weber Christian
0402	Whipple
7100	Disseminated lupus erythematosus
9060	Dog bite
7580	Down's syndrome
1257	Dracontiasis
1257	Dracunculosis
3049	Drug addiction
69230x	eruption, allergic, contact,
69239x	contact type NOS
69501x	fixed drug eruption
69231x	irritant contact
69507x	lichenoid eruption
69232x	photodermatitis
69509x	systemic NOS
3703	Dryness, conjunctiva (see also Sjogrens disease 7102)
5277	mouth

20

702x1x	Dubreuilh's melanosis circumscripta
7286	Dupuytren's contracture
75640x	Dyschondroplasia with hemangiomata
74382x	Dyschromatosis, symmetrical
74382x	universalis
70580x	Dysidrosis
70580x	Dysidrotic eczema
216x03	Dyskeratoma warty
702x3x	Dyskeratosis, Bowenoid
757310	congenita
7560	Dysostosis mandibulofacial
7868	Dysphagia
7565	Dysplasia chondroectodermal
757333	ectodermal, anidrotic
757333	hidrotic
7565	epiphyseal punctate
7565	fibrous polyostotic
75981x	oculoauricularvertebral
2738	Dysproteinemia
7438	Dystrophy dermatochondrocorneal
3598	Gower's muscular
70389x	nail acquired, NOS
75759x	congenital
70988x	Ear piercing granuloma
9249	Ecchymosis
17396x	Eccrine carcinoma
216x22	hidrocystoma
216x22	nevus
216x22	poroma
216x22	spiradenoma
1229	Echinococcosis
68682x	Ecthyma
0512	contagiosum (orf)
68601x	gangrenosum
757333	Ectodermal dysplasia congenital
69512x	Ectodermosis erosiva pluriorificialis
3741	Ectropion
69299x	Eczema NOS
690	asteatotic
69180x	atopic
69289x	contact, NOS
	allergic
69230x	due to drug
69240x	other chemical product
69280x	other specified agent except plants
69260x	plant

69231x	Eczema, contact, irritant, due to drug
69241x	other chemical product
69281x	other specified agent except plants
69261x	plant
	reaction type unspecified
69239x	due to drug
69249x	other chemical product
69289x	other specified agent except plants
69269x	plant
690	craquelé
69290x	discoid
70580x	dyshidrotic
69180x	flexural
69294x	hand NOS
0540	herpeticum
4541	hypostatic
69180x	infantile
690	infective
69830x	lichenified
1103	marginatum due to fungus infection
69290x	nummular
690	seborrheic
69271x	solar
4541	stasis
99901x	vaccinatum
4541	varicose
69293x	Eczematide
9951	Edema angioneurotic
2776	hereditary
4571	lymphatic
7570	Milroy
7823	stasis
7823	NOS or NEC
70388x	Egg shell nails
75680x	Ehlers Danlos syndrome
70181x	Elastic skin, acquired
75680x	congenital
757335	Elastoma juvenile
70116x	perforating
70180x	Elastosis actinic
70282x	nodular with cysts and comedones
70116x	perforans (Miescher)
4579	Elephantiasis, acquired, NOS
7570	congenital
1259	filarial
4579	nostras
4570	postmastectomy
4579	streptococcal
4579	tuberculous

22

7565	Ellis van Creveld syndrome
4449	Embolism
9988	Emphysema surgical
75961x	Encephalofacial angiomatosis
75961x	Encephalocutaneous angiomatosis
4449	Endarteritis, embolic
4449	infective
0939	syphilitic
0178	tuberculous
4249	Endocarditis
228x2x	Endothelioma benign
17190x	malignant
5790	Enteropathy gluten
5798	protein losing
3740	Entropion
70987x	Eosinophilic cellulitis
2778	granuloma
709000	Ephelides
70620x	Epidermal cyst
69511x	Epidermal necrolysis toxic (Lyell)
216x40	Epidermal nevus
757317	Epidermodysplasia verruciformis
757320	Epidermolysis, bullosa
757320	Cockayne
757320	dystrophic
757320	lethal
757320	Pasini
757320	simple
1109	Epidermophytosis, NOS
1100	hair (not favus)
11080x	ide eruption
1106	kerion
1101	nail
1105	skin
7595	Epiloia
3752	Epiphora
216x10	Epithelioma, adenoides cysticum
17390x	basal cell
17394x	basisquamous
216x11	benign calcifying of Malherbe
2329	Borst Jadassohn
216x04	multiple self-healing
17394x	pseudoglandular
17391x	squamous cell
2104	Epulis
024	Equinia
9882	Ergotism
1122	Erosio interdigitalis blastomycetica
919	Erosion of skin

1269	Eruption, creeping
69230x	drug, contact allergic
69231x	irritant
69239x	type unspecified
69501x	fixed
69232x	photodermatitis
	systemic — see type
69509x	NOS
70983x	Hutchinson's summer
11080x	ide eruption due to fungus infection
0540	Kaposi's varicelliform due to herpes simplex
99901x	vaccinia
70912x	pigmented purpuric
69274x	polymorphous light
1269	sandworm
69500x	toxic
216x22	Eruptive hidradenoma
035	Erysipelas
0271	Erysipeloid
69270x	Erythema ab igne
69502x	annulare (Darier)
0239	brucella
69504x	chronicum migrans
69505x	dyschromicum perstans
69580x	elevatum diutinum
69502x	figuratum perstans
69506x	gyratum perstans
69506x	repens
69521x	induratum nontuberculous (Whitfield)
01711x	tuberculous (Bazin)
0570	infectiosum
1103	marginatum due to fungus infection
69502x	rheumaticum
5291	migrans
69510x	multiforme
6910	napkin
69520x	nodosum, not due to sarcoid or tuberculosis
135x2x	due to sarcoidosis
01710x	due to tuberculosis
03080x	leprosum
69503x	palmar
69271x	solar
69500x	toxic
7788	neonatorum
0390	Erythrasma
69298x	Erythroderma, exfoliative
75712x	ichthyosiform congenital
69610x	psoriatic
757316	Erythrokeratodermia variabilis

44381x	Erythromelalgia
5287	Erythroplasia, buccal
2335	of Queyrat
27713x	Erythropoietic protoporphyria
69297x	Erythrose peribuccale pigmentaire (Brocq)
0855	Espundia
0991	Esthiomene
1160	European blastomycosis
7821	Exanthem, NOS or NEC
048	Boston
048	epidemic with meningitis
0578	subitum
0579	viral NOS or NEC
74381x	Excess skin of eyelid, congenital
3748	acquired
918	Excoriation, NOS
69841x	neurotic
69584x	Exfoliation
69298x	Exfoliative, dermatitis
69298x	erythroderma
213x0x	Exostosis, subungual
69580x	Extracellular cholesterolosis
2120	Extranasal glioma

27270x	Fabry's disease
2726	Facial lipodystrophy
3591	Facioscapulohumeral myopathy
2700	Fanconi's syndrome
2729	Farber's disease
024	Farcy
7287	Fasciitis, nodular
27281x	Fat necrosis
7781	neonatal
7425	Faun tail
690	Fausse teigne amiantacée
11081x	Favus
7141	Felty's syndrome
7806	Fever NOS
0783	cat scratch
0360	cerebrospinal
061	dengue
002	enteric
075	glandular
4779	hay
065	hemorrhagic (arthropod borne)
0230	Malta
0830	Q
390	rheumatic

25

0820	Fever, Rocky Mountain spotted
0660	sandfly
114	San Joaquin
0271	swine
0239	undulant
0231	abortus
0230	Malta
0239	NOS
7806	of unknown origin
2866	Fibrinolytic purpura
2770	Fibrocystic disease
21594x	Fibroepithelial tumor of Pinkus
216x52	Fibroma, of skin
21590x	periungual
21590x	ungual
21596x	Fibromatosis, juvenile digital
17191x	Fibrosarcoma
7092	Fibrosis of skin
21595x	Fibrous papule of nose
22994x	Fibroxanthoma, atypical
0570	Fifth disease
1259	Filariasis, NOS
5650	Fissure, anal
5295	Fissured tongue, acquired
7501	congenital
7444	Fistula, auricular
5227	dental
5651	in ano
68689x	to skin NOS
69501x	Fixed drug eruption
9194	Flea bite
7826	Flushing
69443x	Fogo selvagem
70131x	Focal dermal hypoplasia
70131x	Follicular atrophoderma
2648	keratosis due to vitamin A deficiency
2020	lymphoma
704014	mucinosis
70482x	Folliculitis, abscedens et suffodiens
70482x	decalvans
70480x	irritant
7051	miliarial
6809	pyococcal
70183x	ulerythematosa reticulata
216x10	Folliculoma of skin
75080x	Fordyce condition of mouth
75281x	genitalia
70988x	Foreign body granuloma NOS
0578	Fourth disease

26

70583x	Fox disease
70583x	Fox Fordyce disease
75745x	Fragilitas crinum
70388x	unguium
1029	Frambesia
709000	Freckle
702x1x	senile of Hutchinson
0991	Frei's disease
3529	Frey's syndrome
9490	Friction burn
70988x	Friction granuloma
9913	Frostbite
1109	Fungus disease, NOS
1104	foot
1100	hair (not favus)
11080x	ide eruption
1106	kerion
1101	nail
1105	skin
75752x	Furrowing of nails, congenital
70382x	transverse (Beau's lines)
6829	Furuncle

7274	Ganglion
2258	Ganglioneuroma
1025	Gangosa
7854	Gangrene, NOS
4402	arteriosclerotic
7070	decubitus
2507	diabetic
0400	gas
68601x	Meleney's
28660x	Gangrenous purpura
21132x	Gardner's syndrome
27750x	Gargoylism
0400	Gas gangrene
27241x	Gaucher's disease
69882x	Generalised pruritus
0541	Genital herpes
5291	Geographical tongue
0569	German measles
69690x	Gianotti Crosti syndrome
4465	Giant cell arteritis
216x33	pigmented nevus
9951	urticaria
0071	Giardiasis
5231	Gingival hypertrophy
024	Glanders

27

075	Glandular fever
2120	Glioma extranasal
228x1x	Glomangioma
228x1x	Glomus tumor
5290	Glossitis
5296	Glossodynia
7565	Goldenhar's syndrome
6923	Gold eruption
0989	Gonorrhea, NOS
0985	arthritis
0980	balanitis
0981	chordee
0984	conjunctivitis
70912x	Gougerot Blum syndrome
44780x	trisymptome
1026	Goundou
2749	Gout
3598	Gower's panatrophy
21592x	Granular cell myoblastoma
17191x	malignant
00670x	Granuloma, amebic
69581x	annulare
99930x	BCG
70988x	beryllium
11220x	candidal
114	coccidioidal
70984x	disciformis (Miescher)
70988x	ear piercing
2778	eosinophilic
68602x	faciale
70988x	foreign body
70988x	friction
0992	inguinale
70988x	lipophagic
1106	Majocchi's
4463	malignant
4463	midline
69582x	multiforme (Leiker)
70988x	oil
6861	pyogenic
70988x	sea urchin
70988x	silica
70986x	staphylococcal
0311	swimming pool
70988x	talc
6861	telangiectaticum
0992	venereum
4464	Wegener
70988x	zirconium

2881	Granulomatous disease (Good)
70584x	Granulosis rubra nasi
7043	Greying of hair
1269	Ground itch
1257	Guinea worm
095	Gumma
6111	Gynecomastia
757336	Gyrate scalp
69534x	Haber's syndrome
757321	Hailey Hailey disease
70489x	Hair abnormality, acquired NOS
75749x	congenital NOS
75744x	Hair follicle nevus
5293	Hairy black tongue
216x31	Hairy pigmented nevus (Becker)
68680x	Hallopeau acrodermatitis continua
70618x	Halogen eruption, bromide
70618x	iodide
709012	Halo nevus
22991x	Hamartoma
69294x	Hand eczema NOS
0743	Hand, foot and mouth disease
2778	Hand Schuller Christian disease
0309	Hansen's disease NOS
75712x	Harlequin fetus
2700	Hartnup disease
4779	Hay fever
228x2x	Hemangioendothelioma, benign
17190x	malignant
228x9x	Hemangioma NOS
17190x	Hemangiopericytoma
17190x	Hemangiosarcoma
9249	Hematoma, traumatic, unspecified
9981	procedural
2750	Hemochromatosis
2860	Hemophilia
28731x	Hemorrhage, petechial
28731x	in skin
70383x	splinter
7760	Hemorrhagic disease of the newborn
4556	Hemorrhoids NOS
2870	Henoch Schoenlein purpura
2776	Hereditary angioedema
4480	Hereditary hemorrhagic telangiectasia
0740	Herpangina
6943	Herpes gestationis
0549	simplex

29

0539	Herpes zoster
99941x	Herxheimer reaction
74380x	Heterochromia
214x1x	Hibernoma
70581x	Hidradenitis suppurativa
216x22	Hidradenoma, clear cell
216x22	eruptive
216x23	papilliferum
216x23	Hidrocystoma
757333	Hidrotic ectodermal dysplasia
7041	Hirsutes, acquired
75741x	congenital (excluding faun tail 7433)
75280x	Hirsuties papillaris penis
216x50	Histiocytoma
2778	Histiocystosis X
115	Histoplasmosis capsulatum
115	duboysii
2019	Hodgkin's disease
2704	Homocystinuria
1268	Hookworm — creeping eruption
3731	Hordoleum
702x0x	Horn, cutaneous
27751x	Hunter syndrome
27750x	Hurler disease
702x1x	Hutchinson's lentigo
70983x	Hutchinson's summer eruption
27282x	Hyalinosis cutis et mucosae
70983x	Hydroa estivale
70983x	vacciniforme
2281	Hygroma, cystic
7808	Hyperidrosis
70111x	Hyperkeratosis climactericum
70115x	follicularis et perifollicularis in cutem penetrans
75715x	palmaris et plantaris
1023	yaws
	Hyperpigmentation — see pigmentation
216x12	Hyperplasia, senile sebaceous
69831x	pseudoepitheliomatous
	Hypersensitivity — see allergy
44383x	Hypertensive ulcer
6111	Hypertrophy, breast
7555	digit
6078	penis
52853x	lip acquired (Melkersson Rosenthal syndrome 35180x)
7448	congenital
7014	scar
5298	tongue
70131x	Hypoplasia, focal dermal
4541	Hypostatic dermatitis

30

704015	Hypotrichosis, acquired
75740x	congenital
30011x	Hysterical anesthesia
70110x	Ichthyosis acquired
75712x	congenita
75712x	fetalis
75712x	follicularis
75712x	hystrix
75712x	lamellar
75713x	Netherton
75719x	NOS
3563	Refsum
75714x	Rud
75710x	vulgaris, dominant
75771x	sex linked
75712x	Ichthyosiform erythroderma
75712x	bullous
75712x	nonbullous
75712x	Sjögren Larsen
1080x	Ide eruption due to fungus infection
9914	Immersion foot
2793	Immunological deficiency disease, NOS
2790	antibody deficiency syndrome agammaglobulinemia
2790	hypogammaglobulinemia
2791	cellular immunity deficiency syndrome
2792	dysimmunoglobulinemia
2790	hypoimmunoglobulinemia
3348	immune disease with ataxia telangiectasia
2791	Wiskott Aldrich syndrome
584	Impetigo contagiosa
6943	herpetiformis
70620x	Inclusion cyst
757322	Incontinentia pigmenti
69180x	Infantile eczema
075	Infectious mononucleosis
690	Infective dermatitis
690	eczema
70481x	Ingrowing hair
7030	nail
704002	Injury to hair, chemical
704001	physical
595	Injury to nail, finger
597	toe
064	Insect bite, nonvenomous
059	venomous
0020x	Insectophobia
9292x	Intertrigo, bacterial
122	candidal

69292x	Intertrigo, eczematous
1103	fungal
69610x	psoriatic
0402	Intestinal lipodystrophy
2713	Intolerance, disaccharide
2329	Intraepidermal epithelioma, Borst Jadassohn
174x0x	Paget breast
1879	genitalia
1740	nipple
2335	Queyrat erythroplasia
70489x	Inverted follicular hyperkeratosis
70618x	Iododerma
	Irradiation — *see radiodermatitis*
69231x	Irritant contact dermatitis, due to drug
69241x	other chemical product
69281x	other specified agent except plant
69261x	plant
44383x	Ischemic ulcer
	Itch, *see pruritus*
1103	Dhobie
1339	grain
1269	ground
1203	swimmers, due to cercaria
69881x	winter
216x34	Ito nevus

7824	Jaundice, NOS or NEC
69273x	Jessner's lymphocytic infiltration
1341	Jiggers
216x37	Junctional nevus
757335	Juvenile elastoma
216x35	melanoma
70983x	spring eruption
22993x	xanthoendothelioma
1027	Juxta-articular nodes

0850	Kala-azar
17191x	Kaposi's idiopathic hemorrhagic sarcoma
17191x	sarcoma
0540	varicelliform eruption due to herpes simplex
99901x	vaccinia
28740x	Kasabach Merritt syndrome
7014	Keloid
70613x	acne
216x04	Keratoacanthoma
70112x	Keratoderma blenorrhagica
70111x	climactericum
75715x	palmoplantar

75712x	Keratolysis exfoliativa
11180x	plantar
11180x	Keratoma plantare sulcatum
70117x	Keratosis arsenical
70112x	blenorrhagica
75715x	circumscripta
757311	follicularis (Darier's disease)
75715x	palmaris et plantaris
757312	pilaris
70113x	punctata
216x00	seborrheic
702x3x	senilis
702x2x	smoker's lip
5287	smoker's palate
702x3x	solar
70114x	stucco
70114x	tar
1100	Kerion
70489x	Kinking of hair
7587	Klinefelter's syndrome
75962x	Klippel Trenaunay Weber syndrome
70489x	Knotting of hair
7287	Knuckle pads
70381x	Koilonychia, acquired
75752x	congenital
0559	Koplik spots
6070	Kraurosis penis
62400x	vulva
260	Kwashiorkor
70115x	Kyrle's disease
9599	Laceration
75712x	Lamellar ichthyosis
7583	de Lange syndrome
1269	Larva migrans
70181x	Lax skin, acquired
75680x	congenital
1342	Leech
4439	Leg ulcer, arterial
2507	diabetic
44383x	hypertensive
17393x	Marjolin
44383x	Martorel
70780x	neuropathic
70780x	perforating
4540	stasis
7079	traumatic
70780x	trophic
4540	varicose

21598x	Leiomyoma single
21597x	multiple
17191x	Leiomyosarcoma
0854	Leishmaniasis, cutaneous American
0852	Asian
0853	Ethiopian
0850	post-Kala-azar
0851	urban
0855	mucocutaneous
75984x	Lentiginosis syndrome
709000	Lentigo, benign
702x1x	malignant
7310	Leontiasis ossium
75984x	Leopard syndrome
11181x	Lepothrix
2581	Leprechaunism
0309	Leprosy, NOS
0303	borderline
03080x	erythema nodosum
0302	indeterminate
0303	intermediate
0300	lepromatous
03081x	Lucio phenomenon
0301	tuberculoid
1000	Leptospirosis
11181x	Leptothrix
2772	Lesch Nyhan syndrome
2025	Letterer Siwe disease
709012	Leukoderma acquisitum centrifugum
2089	Leukemia, NOS
2050	acute, eosinophilic
2040	lymphoblastic
2060	monocytic
2050	myeloblastic
2050	myeloid
2041	chronic lymphatic
2041	lymphocytic
2061	monocytic
2051	myelocytic
2051	myeloid
2026	mast cell
2031	plasma cell
20880x	Leukemia cutis
2888	Leukemoid reaction
702x2x	Leukokeratosis, labial
5287	nicotina palati
70388x	Leukopathia unguium
702x2x	Leukoplakia lip

34

	Leukoplakia, mouth excluding tongue
	penis
.66	tongue
2401x	vulva
1321	Lice, body
1320	head
1322	pubic
27742x	Lichen amyloidosus
70912x	aureus
70185x	myxedematosus
6971	nitidus
6978	obtusus corneus
6970	planopilaris
6970	planus
69507x	due to drug
6970	ruber planus
70100x	sclerosus et atrophicus
01709x	scrophulosorum
69830x	simplex
757319	spinulosus
6978	striatus
6982	urticatus
69830x	Lichenification
69274x	Light eruption, polymorphous
69271x	sensitivity NOS
	see Photodermatitis
216x40	Linear nevus
70382x	Lines, Beau's
5291	Lingua geographica
5293	nigra
5295	plicata
70981x	Lip sucking
2723	Lipoatrophy
25072x	Lipodystrophy, diabetic
2726	generalised progressive
9623	insulin
0402	intestinal
2723	localised facial
2723	neonatal
2723	NOS
2723	Lipogranuloma, sclerosing
2725	Lipogranulomatosis
27280x	Lipoid dermatoarthritis
27282x	proteinosis
2729	Lipoidosis NOS
214x0x	Lipoma
17191x	Liposarcoma
44600x	Livedo nodularis
7821	racemosa

7821	Livedo, reticularis
1252	Loa loa
6954	Lupus erythematosus, chilblain
6954	chronic discoid
6954	discoid
7100	systemic
01709x	Lupus miliaris faciei
135x1x	Lupus pernio
01703x	Lupus vulgaris
69511x	Lyell's syndrome
2893	Lymphadenitis
22992x	Lymphadenosis benigna cutis
4579	Lymphangiectasis
2281	Lymphangioma circumscriptum
2281	localised
17190x	Lymphangiosarcoma
17190x	postmastectomy
6829	Lymphangitis acute
4579	chronic
2040	Lymphatic leukemia, acute
2041	chronic
4579	Lymphedema, acquired
7570	congenital
4570	postmastectomy
69273x	Lymphocytic infiltration of skin (Jessner)
22992x	Lymphocytoma
0991	Lymphogranuloma venereum
20280x	Lymphoma of skin
0783	Lymphoreticulosis, benign
2001	Lymphosarcoma
2019	Hodgkin's
2000	reticulum cell
9914	Maceration of foot
7560	Macrocephaly
52853x	Macrocheilia, acquired
7448	congenital
7555	Macrodactyly
2552	Macrogenitosomia praecox
2733	Macroglobulinemia
5298	Macroglossia, acquired
7501	congenital
6111	Macromastia
7448	Macrostomia
70131x	Macular atrophy
1174	Madura foot
1174	Maduromycosis
75640x	Maffucci's syndrome

,0912x	Majocchi's disease
1106	granuloma
75715x	Mal de Meleda
5799	Malabsorption, NOS
5799	of fat
5799	of protein
1110	Malassezia furfur
216x11	Malherbe's benign calcifying epithelioma
	Malignant — *see under condition*
261	Malnutrition, NOS
260	protein
2692	vitamin NOS
0230	Malta fever
2703	Maple syrup disease
7821	Marble skin
75980x	Marfan's syndrome
75740x	Marie Unna hypotrichosis
17393x	Marjolin's ulcer
44383x	Martorel ulcer
757331	Mast cell disease
2078	leukemia
2385	nevus
2026	sarcoma
757331	Mastocytosis
0559	Measles
0569	German (rubella)
5998	Meatal ulcer
3732	Meibomian cyst, infected
74280x	Melanocytosis, intracranial
74280x	meningeal
216x34	oculocutaneous
709002	Melanoderma *see melanosis and pigmentation*
216x37	Melanoma benign
216x35	juvenile
1729	malignant
709002	Melanosis NOS
2554	Addisonian
709002	chloasma
702x1x	Dubreuilh
3745	eyelid
702x1x	Hutchinson
74280x	neurocutaneous
709007	occupational
3745	ocular
216x34	oculocutaneous
709004	Riehl
709002	senile
709004	tar
709004	toxic

37

709002	Melasma
68601x	Meleney's ulcer
025	Melioidosis
0230	Melitensis febris
35180x	Melkersson Rosenthal syndrome
2500	Mellitus diabetes, NOS
74280x	Meningeal melanosis
216x53	Meningioma, cutaneous
7419	Meningocele
7419	Meningomyelocele
6272	Menopausal flushing
6272	symptoms
6930	Mercury drug eruption
6930	effects
6930	pigmentation
17191x	Mesenchymoma
	Metabolic disorder — *see condition*
709008	Metal pigmentation (*Excludes* mercury and antimony spots)
1982	Metastasis in skin, carcinoma
1982	sarcoma
1982	unknown primary site
757313	Mibelli's angiokeratoma
757315	porokeratosis
44382x	Microangiopathy of skin, diabetic
4466	thrombotic
1108	Microsporon infection of skin
1100	of hair
4463	Midline granuloma
70984x	Miescher's granulomatosis disciformis
5278	Mikulicz' syndrome
7051	Miliaria
70620x	Milium
70931x	colloid
69181x	Milk crust
0511	Milker's nodules
7570	Milroy's disease
1339	Mite dermatitis
75715x	Mljet disease
	Mole — *see nevus*
0780	Molluscum contagiosum
2377	fibrosum
216x04	sebaceum
216x32	Mongolian spot
7580	Mongolism
75743x	Monilethrix
	Moniliasis *see candidiasis*
2060	Monocytic leukemia, acute
2061	chronic, Naegeli
2061	Schilling

38

216x23	Neoplasm, apocrine, nevus
17396x	sweat gland carcinoma
2276	argentaffinoma
2561	arrhenoblastoma benign, female
2570	male
1830	arrhenoblastoma malignant, female
1869	male
22994x	atypical fibroxanthoma
216x37	balloon cell nevus
17390x	basal cell, carcinoma
17390x	epithelioma
17395x	nevus syndrome
17394x	basisquamous cell carcinoma
99930x	BCG granuloma
216x30	blue nevus, benign
1729	malignant
228x3x	blue rubber bleb nevus
2329	Borst Jadassohn epithelioma
5287	Bowen's disease of mouth
2335	of penis
2336	of scrotum
2329	of skin
5287	of tongue
174x1x	breast carcinoma
174x0x	Paget's disease
216x10	Brooke's disease
2002	Burkitt's lymphoma
2002	Burkitt's tumor
07811x	Buschke Lowenstein condyloma
216x11	calcifying epithelioma of Malherbe
2592	carcinoid tumor
17390x	carcinoma, basal cell
17395x	basal cell nevus syndrome
17394x	basisquamous cell
17391x	epidermoid
2329	intraepidermal Borst Jadassohn
174x0x	intraepidermal Paget of breast
1879	intraepidermal Paget of genitalia
2335	intraepidermal Queyrat
1982	metastatic in skin
17391x	squamous cell
17396x	sweat gland
1999	carcinomatosis
1982	in skin
213x1x	chondroma
1709	chondrosarcoma
276	chromaffinoma
216x22	clear cell hidradenoma
07810x	condyloma acuminatum

41

07811x	Neoplasm, condyloma, Buschke Lowenstein
702x0x	cornu cutaneum
216x21	cylindroma benign
17396x	malignant
216x50	dermatofibroma
17191x	dermatofibrosarcoma
216x51	dermoid cyst of skin
216x03	dyskeratoma, warty
702x3x	dyskeratosis, Bowenoid
70988x	ear piercing granuloma
17396x	eccrine carcinoma
216x22	hidrocystoma
216x22	nevus
216x22	poroma
216x22	spiradenoma
757335	elastoma, juvenile
216x10	epithelioma adenoides cysticum
17390x	basal cell
17394x	basisquamous
216x11	benign calcifying of Malherbe
2329	Borst Jadassohn
216x04	multiple self-healing
17394x	pseudoglandular
17391x	squamous cell
2104	epulis
216x22	eruptive hidradenoma
213x0x	exostosis, subungual
2120	extranasal glioma
27270x	Fabry's disease
2729	Farber's disease
21594x	fibroepithelial tumor of Pinkus
216x52	fibroma of skin
21590x	periungual
21590x	subungual
17191x	fibrosarcoma
21595x	fibrous papule of nose
22994x	fibroxanthoma, atypical
2020	follicular lymphoma
216x10	folliculoma of skin
2258	ganglioneuroma
21132x	Gardner's syndrome
2120	glioma, extranasal
228x1x	glomangioma
228x1x	glomus tumour
21592x	granular cell myoblastoma
17191x	malignant
	granuloma — *see Granuloma*
22991x	hamartoma
228x2x	hemangioendothelioma benign

42

17190x	Neoplasm, hemangioendothelioma, malignant
228x9x	hemangioma NOS
17190x	hemangiopericytoma
17190x	hemangiosarcoma
214x1x	hidrocystoma
216x22	hidradenoma clear cell
216x22	eruptive
216x23	papilliferum
216x23	hidrocystoma
216x50	histiocytoma
2778	histiocytosis X
2019	Hodgkin's disease
702x0x	horn, cutaneous
2329	intraepidermal epithelioma, Borst Jadassohn
174x0x	Paget, breast
1879	Paget, genitalia
174x0x	Paget, nipple
2335	Queyrat erythroplasia
216x37	junctional nevus
757335	juvenile elastoma
216x35	melanoma
22993x	xanthoendothelioma
17191x	Kaposi's idiopathic hemorrhagic sarcoma
17191x	sarcoma
7014	keloid
216x04	keratoacanthoma
70117x	keratosis, arsenical
216x00	seborrheic
702x3x	senilis
702x3x	solar
21598x	leiomyoma single
21597x	multiple
17191x	leiomyosarcoma
214x0x	lipoma
17191x	liposarcoma
22992x	lymphadenosis benigna cutis
2281	lymphangioma circumscriptum
2281	localised
17190x	lymphangiosarcoma
17190x	postmastectomy
22992x	lymphocytoma
20280x	lymphoma of skin
0783	lymphoreticulosis, benign
2001	lymphosarcoma
2019	Hodgkin's
2000	reticulum cell
216x11	Malherbe's calcifying epithelioma
757331	mast cell disease
2385	nevus

216x37	Neoplasm, melanoma, benign
216x35	juvenile
1729	malignant
216x53	meningioma, cutaneous
17191x	mesenchymoma
1982	metastasis in skin, carcinoma
1982	sarcoma
1982	unknown primary site
4462	midline granuloma
2377	molluscum fibrosum
216x04	sebaceum
216x04	multiple self-healing epitheliomata
2021	mycosis fungoides
2030	myeloma
21592x	myoblastoma, granular cell
17191x	malignant
216x24	myoepithelioma
2224	myoma, dartoic
17191x	myxosarcoma
2158	neurilemmoma
2158	neurofibroma
2377	multiple
2377	neurofibromatosis
17191x	neurofibrosarcoma
2158	neuroma, digital
2158	traumatic
22993x	nevoxanthoendothelioma
	nevus — *see Nevus*
217	nipple adenoma
213x1x	osteochondroma
70930x	osteoma cutis
174x0x	Paget's disease of breast
174x0x	of nipple
1879	of genitalia
22990x	papilloma, NOS
2158	paraganglionoma
2010	paragranuloma of Hodgkin
21590x	periungual fibroma
2556	pheochromocytoma
216x11	pilomatrixoma
2386	plasmacytoma
21594x	polyp, fibroepithelial
216x22	poroma
2000	reticulocytoma
2000	reticuloendothelioma
22994x	reticulohistiocytoma
2000	reticulosarcoma
2000	reticulum cell sarcoma
21593x	rhabdomyoma

44

17191x	Neoplasm, rhabdomyosarcoma
2012	sarcoma, Hodgkin
17191x	Kaposi
2026	mast cell
2000	reticulum cell
2158	Schwannoma
216x12	sebaceous adenoma
216x12	epithelioma
17396x	gland carcinoma
70621x	sebocystomatosis
216x00	seborrheic wart
216x04	self-healing epithelioma
70186x	skin tags, acquired
216x22	spiradenoma
17391x	squamous cell carcinoma
70621x	steatocystoma multiplex
216x22	sweat gland adenoma
17396x	sweat gland carcinoma
216x23	syringocystadenoma papilliferum
216x20	syringoma
216x10	trichoepithelioma
216x10	trichofolliculoma
216x21	turban tumour
	wart — *see Verruca*
216x03	warty dyskeratoma
75713x	Netherton's syndrome
2158	Neurilemmoma
17191x	Neuroepithelioma
74280x	Neurocutaneous disorders
69180x	Neurodermatitis, diffuse, atopic eczema
69830x	local, lichen simplex
2158	Neurofibroma
2377	multiple
2377	Neurofibromatosis
17191x	Neurofibrosarcoma
2158	Neuroma, digital
2158	Neuroma
70780x	Neuropathic ulcer
3579	Neuropathy, NOS
69841x	Neurotic excoriations
28800x	Neutropenia, cyclical
69513x	Neutrophilic syndrome of Sweet
22993x	Nevoxanthoendothelioma
216x36	Nevus amelanotic
709011	anemicus
44810x	araneus
17395x	basal cell syndrome
216x30	blue
1729	malignant

45

216x37	Nevus, cellular
757318	comedonicus
216x37	compound
216x41	connective tissue
216x41	elasticus
216x40	epidermal
216x34	fuscoceruleus ophthalmomaxillaris
216x33	giant pigmented
75744x	hair follicle
216x31	hairy pigmented (Becker)
709012	halo (Sutton)
216x34	Ito
216x37	junctional
216x40	linear
216x42	lipomatodes superficialis
216x42	lipomatosus
2385	mast cell
216x34	oculocutaneous
75081x	oral (white sponge)
216x34	Ota
216x37	pigmented
228x0x	portwine
216x43	sebaceus (Jadassohn)
216x12	senile sebaceous
44810x	spider
44812x	strawberry
709012	Sutton's
216x23	syringocystadenoma papilliferum
216x40	unius lateris
44892x	vascular NEC or NOS
216x40	verrucous
75081x	white sponge
75744x	woolly hair
27242x	Niemann Pick disease
1040	Njovera
7999	NO DIAGNOSIS MADE
7999	NO DISEASE FOUND
0405	Nocardiosis
7151	Nodes Heberden
0511	milker's
4210	Osler
390	rheumatic
7287	Nodular fasciitis
44780x	vasculitis
1027	Nodules, juxta-articular due to yaws
7140	rheumatoid
2410	thyroid
5281	Noma
1160	North American blastomycosis

13301x	Norwegian scabies
261	Nutrition, deficient NOS
2599	Obesity of endocrine origin, NOS
2780	Obesity, NOS
709007	Occupational pigmentation
70982x	stigma
27023x	Ochronosis
6946	Ocular pemphigus
75981x	Oculoauricular vertebral dysplasia
216x34	Oculocutaneous nevus
36320x	syndrome
75982x	Oculolentodigital dysplasia
	Oedema *see Edema*
70612x	Oil acne
6921	dermatitis
70988x	granuloma
2701	Oligophrenia, phenylpyruvic
68682x	Omphalitis
7510	Omphalomesenteric duct anomaly
1253	Onchocerciasis
1253	Onchodermatitis
68102x	Onychia
70388x	Onychodystrophy, acquired
75752x	congenital
70385x	Onychogryphosis
70384x	Onycholysis
1101	Onychomycosis
70380x	Onychophagy
0663	O'Nyong Nyong
8798	Open wound
75081x	Oral epithelial nevus
757334	Oral facial digital syndrome
6287	Oral florid papillomatosis
1361	Oral genital ulceration
0512	Orf
4851	Oriental sore
480	Osler Weber Rendu disease
210	Osler's nodes
70582x	Osmidrosis
13x1x	Osteochondroma
0930x	Osteoma cutis
682	Osteomalacia
565	Osteo-onychodysplasia
565	Osteopoikilosis
330	Osteoporosis, senile
16x34	Ota's nevus
802	Otitis externa

1119	Otomycosis
1274	Oxyuriasis
4722	Ozena

70187x	Pachyderma
70187x	Pachydermoperiostosis
75750x	Pachyonychia congenita
174x0x	Paget's disease of breast
1879	of genitalia
174x0x	of nipple
1879	of scrotum
28723x	Painful bruising syndrome
75715x	Palmar plantar hyperkeratosis (tylosis)
70111x	(keratoderma climactericum)
3598	Panatrophy of Gowers
7293	Panniculitis
22990x	Papilloma of skin NOS
75715x	Papillon Lefevre syndrome
70185x	Papular mucinosis
6982	urticaria
13300x	Papule, postscabetic
01704x	Papulonecrotic tuberculide
44783x	Papulosis, malignant atrophic (Degos)
1161	Paracoccidioidomycosis
70988x	Paraffinoma
17191x	Paraganglionoma
2010	Paragranuloma of Hodgkin
69622x	Parakeratosis variegata
605	Paraphimosis
69620x	Parapsoriasis en gouttes
69623x	en plaques
69620x	guttate
69620x	lichenoides chronica
69622x	variegata
69621x	varioliformis
30020x	Parasitophobia
7820	Paresthesia
0029	Paratyphoid
68100x	Paronychia, acute
68101x	chronic
70102x	Pasini et Pierini syndrome
757320	Pasini's syndrome
0272	Pasteurella multocida
0209	pestis
0272	septica
021	tularensis
75560x	Patella nail syndrome
1320	Pediculosis capitis

1321	Pediculosis corporis
1322	pubis
2652	Pellagra
6946	Pemphigoid, benign mucous membrane
6945	bullous
6942	juvenile
6946	ocular
6946	scarring
684	Pemphigus, acute
69443x	Brazilian
684	butcher's
757321	chronic familial benign
69440x	erythematosus
69440x	foliaceus
757321	Hailey Hailey
684	neonatorum
69440x	Senear Usher
0900	syphiliticus
69442x	vegetans
69441x	vulgaris
75280x	Penile pearly papules
60782x	plastic induration
70780x	Perforating ulcer
5282	Periadenitis mucosae necrotica recurrens
44600x	Periarteritis nodosa
70482x	Perifolliculitis capitis abscedens
69533x	Perioral dermatitis
21590x	Periungual fibroma
1120	Perleche candidal
68682x	other
9915	Pernio (chilblain)
135x1x	lupus
7827	Petechiae, NOS *see Purpura*
21130x	Peutz Jeghers syndrome
60782x	Peyronie's disease
68682x	Phagedena
99942x	Phenomenon, Arthus
03081x	Lucio (leprosy)
4430	Raynaud
2701	Phenylketonuria
2701	Phenylpyruvic oligophrenia
2556	Pheochromocytoma
605	Phimosis
4549	Phlebectasia, acquired
7476	congenital
4510	Phlebitis of lower extremities
4539	Phlebothrombosis
4531	migratory
4512	Phlegmasia alba dolens

49

69271x	Photodermatitis, NOS
69232x	due to drug
69262x	due to plant
69242x	due to specified agent NEC
	Photosensitivity — see Photodermatitis
2648	Phrynoderma
1322	Phthiriasis
1322	Phthirius pubis
1178	Phycomycosis
69262x	Phytophotodermatitis
27021x	Piebaldism
1113	Piedra, black
1112	white
216x31	Pigmentary hairy nevus (Becker)
	Pigmentation, *see Melanosis or diseases*
709008	hyperpigmentation, arsenical
709008	due to metals except mercury
9850	mercury
709013	postinflammatory
709002	pregnancy
709003	hypopigmentation postinflammatory
709007	occupational
709013	racial (symptomatic)
709009	NOS
216x31	Pigmented hairy nevus
216x37	Pigmented nevus NOS
70912x	Pigmented purpuric eruption
70620x	Pilar cyst
4556	Piles
75743x	Pili annulati
70481x	incarnati
75743x	torti
216x11	Pilomatrixoma
685	Pilonidal abscess
685	cyst
685	dimple
685	sinus
9850	Pink disease
21594x	Pinkus' fibroepithelial tumor
1039	Pinta, NOS
1031	intermediate lesions
1032	late lesions
1033	mixed lesions
1030	primary lesion (chancre)
1274	Pinworms
70387x	Pitting of nails
6965	Pityriasis alba
690	amiantacea
690	capitis

69631x	Pityriasis, circinata
69621x	lichenoides et varioliformis acuta
69620x	lichenoides chronica
1111	nigra
69630x	rosea
69631x	rotunda
6964	rubra pilaris
1110	versicolor
69260x	Plant dermatitis, allergic contact
69261x	irritant contact
69269x	NOS
69262x	light provoked
2031	Plasma cell leukemia
2386	Plasmacytoma
1320	Plica polonica
70913x	Poikiloderma atrophicans vasculare (Jacobi)
70911x	Bloom's
709005	Civatte
757332	congenital
757332	Thomson
69260x	Poison ivy dermatitis
4770	Pollinosis
4463	Polyarteritis granulomatous
44600x	nodosa
7339	Polychondritis relapsing
2384	Polycythemia vera
2890	secondary
7550	Polydactyly
7287	Polyfibromatosis syndrome
2589	Polyglandular syndrome
75715x	Polykeratosis of Touraine
7576	Polymastia
69274x	Polymorphous light eruption
725	Polymyalgia rheumatica
7565	Polyostotic fibrous dysplasia
21594x	Polyp, fibroepithelial, Pinkus
21131x	Polyposis coli
70580x	Pompholyx
757315	Porokeratosis of Mibelli
216x22	Poroma
27714x	Porphyria, acquired
27710x	congenital erythropoietic
27711x	cutanea tarda
27713x	erythropoietic protoporphyria
27711x	hepatic
27719x	hereditary NOS
27714x	secondary
27714x	toxic
27712x	variegata

51

228x0x	Portwine nevus
13300x	Postscabetic papules
4570	Postmastectomy lymphedema
17190x	lymphosarcoma
4591	Postphlebitic syndrome
7441	Preauricular appendage
7444	sinus
702x9x	Precancerous dermatosis, NOS
709002	Pregnancy chloasma
6468	eruption
709002	pigmentation
6465	pruritus (excluding herpes gestationis 6943)
2021	Premycotic eruption
2021	Prereticulotic eruption
7070	Pressure sore
7070	ulcer
24680x	Pretibial myxedema
7051	Prickly heat
69260x	Primula dermatitis
7595	Pringle's disease
2598	Progeria
5799	Protein malabsorption
260	malnutrition
27282x	Proteinosis, lipoid
27713x	Protoporphyria, erythropoietic
1368	Protothecosis
69180x	Prurigo, Besnier
70983x	estivale
69832x	nodularis
3053	psychogenic
6465	pregnancy
6980	Pruritus, ani
25070x	diabetic
69882x	generalised
6465	pregnancy (excluding herpes gestationis 6943)
3063	psychogenic
6981	scroti
69880x	senile
6981	vulvae
757302	Pseudo-acanthosis nigricans
69831x	Pseudo-epitheliomatous hyperplasia
17394x	Pseudo-glandular epithelioma
704013	Pseudopelade
757300	Pseudoxanthoma elasticum
69610x	Psoriasis, NOS
6960	arthropathic
69610x	erythrodermic
69612x	pustular, generalised
69611x	of palms and soles

70388x	Pterygium of nail
70113x	Punctate keratosis
7806	P U O
2870	Purpura, allergic
2870	anaphylactoid
70912x	annularis telangiectoides
28724x	carbromal
2732	cryoglobulinemic
2866	fibrinolytic
28660x	fulminans
28660x	gangrenous
2870	Henoch Schoenlein
2730	hyperglobulinemic
2879	idiopathic
2733	macroglobulinemic
0360	meningococcal
2870	nonthrombocytopenic
28720x	pigmented
28722x	rheumatic
267	scorbutic
2875	sedormid
28725x	senile
28720x	stasis
28725x	steroid
2874	thrombocytopenic
4466	thrombotic
28722x	toxic
28721x	traumatic
6948	Pustular bacterid
69612x	psoriasis, generalised
69611x	of palms and soles
6948	Pustulosis palmaris et plantaris
6941	subcorneal (Sneddon Wilkinson disease)
68609x	Pyoderma, NOS
68602x	chancriform
68600x	gangrenosum
68601x	vegetans
6861	Pyogenic granuloma
7806	Pyrexia of unknown origin
0830	Q fever
2335	Queyrat's erythroplasia
69282x	Radiodermatitis
69282x	Radionecrosis
69260x	Ragweed dermatitis
5276	Ranula

6910	Rash, diaper
69230x	drug contact allergic
69231x	irritant
	systemic, *see type*
6910	napkin
7089	nettle, NOS
4430	Raynaud's disease
4430	phenomenon
4430	syndrome
	Reaction, allergic — see Allergy
	drug — see type
99941x	Herxheimer
2888	leukemoid
99940x	serum
99943x	Shwartzmann
2377	Recklinghausen's disease of nerves
3563	Refsum's syndrome
0993	Reiter's disease
7339	Relapsing polychondritis
4480	Rendu Osler Weber syndrome
2000	Reticuloendothelioma
22994x	Reticulohistiocytoma
2000	Reticulosarcoma
20280x	Reticulosis of skin NOS
69583x	Reticulosis, lipomelanic
2000	Reticulum cell sarcoma
21593x	Rhabdomyoma
17191x	Rhabdomyosarcoma
390	Rheumatic node
7140	Rheumatoid arteritis
7148	Rheumatoid nodule
1177	Rhinophycomycosis
69532x	Rhinophyma
0401	Rhinoscleroma
1170	Rhinosporidiosis
69260x	Rhus dermatitis
2660	Riboflavin deficiency
0832	Rickettsial pox
709004	Riehl's melanosis
74280x	Riley Day syndrome
75743x	Ringed hair
1100	Ringworm, hair
11080x	ide eruption
1106	kerion
1101	nail
1109	NOS
1108	skin
1105	Tokelau
0820	Rocky Mountain spotted fever

17390x	Rodent ulcer
69530x	Rosacea
69531x	Rosaceous conjunctivitis
69531x	keratitis
0271	Rosenbach's erysipeloid
0578	Roseola infantum
0913	syphilitic
70781x	Rot, Barcoo
7293	Rothman Makai syndrome
757332	Rothmund Thomson syndrome
0569	Rubella
75714x	Rud's syndrome

70101x	Sabre, coup de
0905	tibia
2102	Salivary gland adenoma
757330	de Sanctis Cacchione syndrome
0660	Sandfly fever
1269	Sandworm eruption
114	San Joaquin valley fever
135x0x	Sarcoid NOS
135x0x	Sarcoidosis NOS
135x0x	Darier Roussy
135x2x	erythema nodosum syndrome
135x1x	lupus pernio
135x0x	miliary
1982	Sarcoma, in skin, NOS
2012	Hodgkin
17191x	Kaposi
2001	lymphoblastic
2001	lymphocytic
2026	mast cell
2000	reticulum cell
1982	Sarcomatosis, in skin alone and other tissues
13300x	Scabies (human)
13302x	animal
13301x	Norwegian
13300x	postscabietic papules
757337	Scalp defect, congenital
7092	Scar, NOS
7092	adherent
7014	hypertrophic
7014	keloidal
7092	painful
0341	Scarlet fever
70912x	Schamberg disease
1203	Schistosome dermatitis
1203	granuloma

2158	Schwannoma
70131x	Schweninger Buzzi anetoderma
71080x	Scleredema
7781	Sclerema
7101	Scleroderma, diffuse
70101x	localised
7101	systemic
7180	Sclerodermatomyositis
70185x	Scleromyxedema
7293	Sclerosing lipogranuloma
7101	Sclerosis, systemic
7595	tuberous
01702x	Scrofuloderma
5295	Scrotal tongue
267	Scurvy
70988x	Sea urchin granuloma
216x12	Sebaceous adenoma
17396x	carcinoma
70620x	cyst
216x12	epithelioma
17396x	gland carcinoma
7069	disease, NOS
216x43	nevus (Jadassohn)
70621x	Sebocystomatosis
7063	Seborrhea
690	Seborrheic dermatitis
690	eczema
216x00	keratosis
216x00	wart
69293x	Seborrheide
1982	Secondary neoplasm in skin NOS
2875	Sedormid purpura
216x04	Self healing epithelioma
69840x	Self mutilation
69440x	Senear Usher syndrome
228x9x	Senile angioma
69296x	dermatitis
70180x	elastosis
702x3x	keratosis
69880x	pruritus
28725x	purpura
216x12	sebaceous adenoma
216x12	hyperplasia
7820	Sensation, burning
5296	burning tongue
7820	Sensation, prickling
7820	Sense loss
28733x	Sensitisation, autoerythrocyte
69291x	dermatitis

	Sensitivity, *see Allergy*
	Sepsis of skin, *see Abscess*
0389	Septicemia NOS
99940x	Serum reaction
9995	sickness
7588	Sex chromosome anomaly NOS
2022	Sézary syndrome
70388x	Shedding of nails
0539	Shingles
69280x	Shoe dermatitis
99943x	Shwartzmann reaction
2825	Sickle cell anemia
9995	Sickness serum
70988x	Silica granuloma
5227	Sinus, dental
685	dermal
685	pilonidal
7444	preauricular
7444	thyroglossal
68689x	NOS or NEC
7102	Sjögren syndrome
70186x	Skin tags (acrochordon)
68682x	Sloughing skin
0509	Smallpox, NOS
0500	major
0501	minor
702x2x	Smoker's keratosis, lip
5287	palate
9062	Snake bite, non-venomous
9050	venomous
6941	Sneddon Wilkinson disease
0990	Soft chancre
700	Soft corn
70388x	Soft nails
0990	Soft sore
0851	Sore Delhi
70781x	desert
5289	mouth, denture
0851	Sore, Delhi
7070	pressure
0990	soft
70782x	tropical
70781x	veldt
9051	Spider bite, venomous
44810x	Spider nevus
7561	Spina bifida occulta
216x22	Spiradenoma
70388x	Splitting of nails
70381x	Spoon nails

1171	Sporotrichosis
70131x	Spots, atrophic
709001	café au lait
44811x	Campbell de Morgan
0559	Koplik
216x32	Mongolian
0360	Spotted fever, meningococcal
0820	Rocky Mountain
70983x	Spring eruption
5791	Sprue
7269	Spur, calcaneal
17391x	Squamous cell carcinoma
17391x	epithelioma
228x0x	Stain, portwine
4541	Stasis dermatitis
4541	eczema
7823	edema due to varicose veins
2830x	purpura
4540	ulcer
70621x	Steatocystoma multiplex
5798	Steatorrhea
2563	Stein Leventhal syndrome
70617x	Steroid acne
70132x	atrophy
70132x	striae
69512x	Stevens Johnson syndrome
7143	Still's disease
9059	Stings, venomous NOS
9985	Stitch abscess
5282	Stomatitis, aphthous
1120	candidal
101	Vincent's
2669	vitamin deficiency
44812x	Strawberry mark nevus
70130x	Striae albicantes
70130x	atrophicae
70130x	distensae
70132x	steroid
70114x	Stucco keratosis
75961x	Sturge Weber syndrome
3731	Stye
4210	Subacute bacterial endocarditis
6941	Subcorneal pustular dermatosis
6941	pustulosis
27281x	Subcutaneous fat necrosis
213x0x	Subungual exostosis
21590x	fibroma
69275x	Sunburn
7550	Supernumerary digit

7576	Supernumerary nipple
709012	Sutton's disease
709012	nevus
5282	periadenitis mucosae necrotica recurrens
5282	ulcer
216x23	Sweat gland adenoma, apocrine
216x22	eccrine
216x29	NOS
17396x	carcinoma
69513x	Sweet's acute neutrophilic syndrome
1203	Swimmer's itch
0311	Swimming pool granuloma
0271	Swine fever
7551	Syndactyly
2552	Syndrome, Achard Thiers
7565	Albright (polyostotic fibrous dysplasia)
2791	Aldrich Wiskott
709010	Alezzandrini
7560	Apert
70185x	Arndt Gottron
17395x	basal cell nevus
9598	battered baby
1361	Behçet
757322	Bloch Sulzberger
70911x	Bloom
75983x	Bonnet Dechaume Blanc
7043	Book
7565	Buschke Ollendorf
2782	Caffey
2592	carcinoid
2882	Chediak Higashi
25801x	Cockayne, dwarfism
757320	epidermolysis bullosa
7583	Cornelia de Lange
2774	Crigler Najjar
21133x	Cronkhite Canada
7101	CRST
2550	Cushing
75680x	Danlos Ehlers
7583	de Lange
757330	Sanctis Cacchione
7580	Down
75680x	Ehlers Danlos
7565	Ellis van Creveld
2700	Fanconi
7141	Felty
3529	Frey
21132x	Gardner
69690x	Gianotti Crosti

7565	Syndrome, Goldenhar
70912x	Gougerot Blum
3598	Gowers
69534x	Haber
2778	Hand Schuller Christian
2870	Henoch Schoenlein
27751x	Hunter
27750x	Hurler
28740x	Kasabach Merritt
7587	Klinefelter
75962x	Klippel Trenaunay Weber
75984x	lentiginosis
75984x	leopard
2772	Lesch Nyhan
69511x	Lyell
75640x	Maffucci
75980x	Marfan
35180x	Melkersson Rosenthal
5278	Mikulicz
27752x	Morquio Brailsford
2061	Naegeli
75560x	Nail patella
75713x	Netherton
69513x	neutrophilic of Sweet
36320x	oculocutaneous
757334	oral facial digital
28733x	painful bruising
75715x	Papillon Lefevre
757320	Pasini
70102x	Pasini et Pierini
75570x	Patella — nail
21130x	Peutz Jegher
7287	polyfibromatosis
2589	polyglandular
4591	postphlebitic
4430	Raynaud's
3563	Refsum
0993	Reiter
4480	Rendu Osler Weber
74280x	Riley Day
7293	Rothman Makai
757332	Rothmund Thomson
75714x	Rud
757330	Sanctis Cacchione
69440x	Senear Usher
2022	Sézary
7102	Sjögren
2563	Stein Leventhal
69512x	Stevens Johnson

75961x	Syndrome, Sturge Weber
69513x	Sweet
7101	Thibierge Weissenbach
757332	Thomson
75715x	Thost Unna
7586	Turner
36321x	Vogt Koyanagi
27021x	Waardenberg
0363	Waterhouse Friderichsen
7293	Weber Christian
4463	Wegener
2598	Werner
2791	Wiskott Aldrich
70386x	yellow nail
7275	Synovial cyst
21591x	Synovioma
0913	Syphilide
0979	Syphilis, NOS
0909	congenital
0929	latent
0911	primary, anal
0910	genital
0912	other
0913	secondary
0971	sero-positive
30021x	Syphilophobia
216x23	Syringocystadenoma papilliferum
216x20	Syringoma
3360	Syringomyelia
7100	Systemic lupus erythematosus
7101	sclerosis

0942	Tabes dorsalis
0941	Taboparesis
70186x	Tag skin — acquired
28731x	Talon noir
17392x	Tar epithelioma
70114x	keratosis
709004	melanosis
709004	pigmentation
709006	Tattoo
44890x	Telangiectasia, NOS
44890x	arborising
3348	ataxia
44890x	essential
44890x	generalised
4480	hereditary hemorrhagic
757331	macularis eruptiva perstans

61

44890x	Telangiectasia, primary
44810x	spider
704011	Telogen effluvium
4464	Temporal arteritis
7101	Thibierge Weissenbach syndrome
757332	Thomson's disease
75715x	Thost Unna
1274	Threadworm
4431	Thromboangiitis obliterans
2871	Thrombocythemia
2874	Thrombocytopenia, idiopathic
2791	Aldrich Wiskott
28750x	Kasabach Merritt
4465	thrombotic
4510	Thrombophlebitis of lower legs
4531	migrans
4465	Thrombocytic thrombocytopenia
11222x	Thrush, cutaneous
11220x	granulomatous
11221x	mucocutaneous chronic
1120	oral
11222x	perineal
744	Thyroglossal cyst
744	duct
744	sinus
9064	Tick bite
690	Tinea amiantacea
1100	capitis
1105	corporis
1103	cruris
1105	imbricata
1102	manuum
1111	nigra
1104	pedis
1101	unguium
1110	versicolor
1109	NOS
7030	Toenail, ingrowing
1105	Tokelau ringworm
2748	Tophus of skin
1174	Torulosis
69511x	Toxic epidermal necrolysis
69500x	eruption
6468	of pregnancy
69500x	erythema
7788	neonatorum
1280	Toxocariasis
130	Toxoplasmosis
9914	Trench foot

101	Trench mouth
124	Trichinosis
216x10	Trichoepithelioma
216x10	Trichofolliculoma
1319	Trichomoniasis
11183x	Trichomycosis
11181x	Trichonocardiosis
75745x	Trichonodosis
75745x	Trichorrhexis nodosa
75743x	Trichostasis spinulosa
704000	Trichotillomania
1273	Trichuriasis
7580	Trisomy 21
44780x	Trisymptome of Gougerot and Blum
1338	Trombiculosis
70780x	Trophic ulcer
9914	Tropical maceration of feet
5791	Tropical sprue
70782x	Tropical ulcer
0865	Trypanosomiasis African
0862	American
01709x	Tuberculide, NOS
0176	Tuberculosis, Addison's disease
01711x	Bazin's disease
01705x	cold abscess in skin
01710x	erythema nodosum
01703x	lupus vulgaris
0189	miliary
01704x	papulonecrotic tuberculide
01700x	primary ulcer of skin
01702x	scrophuloderma
01701x	verrucosa cutis
7595	Tuberous sclerosis
021	Tularemia
1340	Tumbu fly myiasis
	Tumour, *see neoplasm*
1341	Tungiasis
216x21	Turban tumor, benign
17396x	malignant
7586	Turner's syndrome
75715x	Tylosis
0020	Typhoid
080	Typhus
7079	Ulcer, NOS
4781	ala nasi
00670x	amebic of skin
5282	aphthous

4402	Ulcer, arteriosclerotic
0311	Buruli
0854	chiclero
7079	chronic NOS
7070	decubitus
0328	diphtheritic
44383x	hypertensive
17393x	Marjolin
44383x	Martorel
5998	meatal
68601x	Meleney
0319	mycobacterial (excluding tuberculosis)
70780x	neuropathic
1361	oral genital
17390x	rodent
4540	stasis
5282	Sutton's
0910	syphilitic, primary
0913	secondary
70780x	trophic
70782x	tropical
01700x	tuberculous, primary
4540	varicose
4540	venous
6165	vulval, aphthous
70184x	Ulerythema ophryogenes
7999	Undiagnosed disease
0239	Undulant fever
7537	Urachus cyst
27282x	Urbach's lipoid proteinosis
5993	Urethral caruncle
7089	Urticaria, NOS
70881x	acute NOS
9951	angioneurotic
70882x	aquagenic
70880x	chronic
7082	cold
9951	giant
7082	heat
6982	papular
757331	pigmentosa
70831x	pressure
69271x	solar

99900x	Vaccinia, accidental
0510	acquired from cow
99901x	eczema vaccinatum
99903x	gangrenosa

64

99902x	Vaccinia, generalised
99900x	localised accidental
0510	acquired from cow
99904x	NEC (complication of vaccination)
99909x	NOS (complication of vaccination)
1321	Vagabond's disease
052	Varicella
4541	Varicose dermatitis
4541	eczema
4510	phlebitis
4540	ulcer
4549	veins
4549	Varix
0500	Variola major
0501	minor
44780x	Vasculitis allergic
44780x	cutaneous
44600x	disseminated
4464	giant cell
44780x	hypersensitivity
44780x	leukocytoclastic
44601x	necrotising
44780x	nodular
44780x	purpuric
70781x	Veldt sore
9050	Venomous bite of snake, or reptile
9051	spider
07811x	Verruca acuminata
70117x	arsenical
01701x	necrogenic
6880	Peruvian
216x00	seborrheic
702x3x	solare
07810x	viral
07810x	vulgaris
0880	Verruga peruana
101	Vincent's angina
2552	Virilism
0799	Virus infection, NOS
2692	Vitamin deficiency, NOS
709010	Vitiligo
36321x	Vogt Koyanagi syndrome
2377	von Recklinghausen's disease of nerves
6241	Vulval atrophy
6161	Vulvitis
27021x	Waardenberg's syndrome
70117x	Wart, arsenical

07810x	Wart, common, *see verruca*
07810x	filiform
216x02	Murray Williams
0880	Peruvian
07810x	plane
07810x	plantar
216x00	seborrheic
702x3x	solar
07810x	viral
216x03	Warty dyskeratoma
9053	Wasp sting
0363	Waterhouse Friderichsen syndrome
3804	Wax in ear
7551	Webbed fingers
7445	neck
7551	toes
7293	Weber Christian disease
4463	Wegener's granuloma
4463	granulomatosis
70620x	Wen
2598	Werner's syndrome
9914	Wet feet syndrome
0402	Whipple's disease
27021x	White forelock disease
70620x	Whitehead
75081x	White sponge nevus
68100x	Whitlow, NOS
0546	herpetic
1728	melanotic
0912	syphilitic
69881x	Winter itch
2791	Wiskott Aldrich syndrome
75744x	Woolly hair nevus
1257	Worm, Guinea
8798	Wound, open
7828	Wrinkles

27210x	Xanthelasma
22993x	Xanthoendothelioma, juvenile
22993x	Xanthogranuloma
27219x	Xanthoma, NOS
25073x	Xanthoma diabeticorum
27212x	eruptive
27219x	Xanthomatosis, NOS
27211x	systemic
70110x	Xeroderma, acquired
757314	congenital
757330	pigmentosum

2640	Xerophthalmia
5277	Xerostomia congenital
69282x	Xray dermatitis
69282x	necrosis

1029	Yaws, NOS
1020	chancre
1021	crab
1022	early
1023	hyperkeratosis
1027	juxta-articular nodes
1026	late
70386x	Yellow nail syndrome

70988x	Zirconium granuloma
60784x	Zoon's balanitis
0539	Zoster, herpes

Diagnoses Listed in Numerical Order

I   **Infective and Parasitic Diseases**

0067   Amebic infection of other sites
            00670x Ameboma of skin
0170   Tuberculosis of skin and subcutaneous cellular tissue
            01700x Primary tuberculous ulcer of skin
            01701x Necrogenic wart
                    Tuberculosis verrucosa cutis
            01702x Scrophuloderma
            01703x Lupus vulgaris
            01704x Papulonecrotic tuberculide
            01705x Cold abscess in skin
            01709x Other and unspecified tuberculides
                    includes: acnitis
                            lichen scrophulosorum
                            lupus miliaris faciei
0171   Erythema nodosum with hypersensitivity reaction in tuberculosis
            01710x Erythema nodosum due to tuberculosis
            01711x Bazin's disease
                    Erythema induratum due to tuberculosis
0308   Leprosy NEC
            03080x Erythema nodosum leprosum
            03081x Lucio phenomenon in leprosy
0781   Viral warts
            07810x Viral warts excluding genital warts
            07811x Buschke Lowenstein condyloma
                    Condylomata acuminata
1108   Dermatophytosis of other sites
            11080x Id (or ide) eruption due to fungus infection
            11081x Favus
1118   Other dermatomycosis
            11180x Keratolysis
                    Keratoma plantare sulcatum
            11181x Lepothrix
                    Leptothrix
                    Trichonocardiosis
            11182x Acladiosis
            11183x Trichomycosis
1122   Candidiasis of skin
            11220x Candidal granuloma

	11221x Chronic mucocutaneous candidiasis
	11222x Candidiasis of skin NOS
1330	Scabies

        11221x Chronic mucocutaneous candidiasis
        11222x Candidiasis of skin NOS
1330   Scabies
        13300x Scabies — human
                includes: post-scabetic papules
                        post-scabetic pruritus
                excludes: Norwegian scabies
        13301x Norwegian scabies
        13302x Animal scabies in man
                includes: cat scabies
                        dog scabies
135   Sarcoidosis
        135x0x Sarcoidosis of skin and other tissues
                includes: Boeck's sarcoid
                        Darier Roussy sarcoid
                        miliary sarcoid
                        sarcoid NOS
                        sarcoidosis NOS
                excludes: Besnier's lupus pernio
                        erythema nodosum due to sarcoidosis
        135x1x Besnier's lupus pernio
                Lupus pernio
        135x2x Erythema nodosum due to sarcoidosis

II   Neoplasms

1719   Malignant neoplasm of connective and other soft tissue, site
        unspecified
        17190x Vascular neoplasm
                includes: angioendothelioma
                        angiosarcoma
                        hemangioendothelioma
                        hemangiopericytoma
                        hemangiosarcoma
                        lymphangiosarcoma
        17191x Nonvascular neoplasm
                includes: dermatofibrosarcoma
                        fibrosarcoma
                        Kaposi's idiopathic hemorrhagic sarcoma
                        leiomyosarcoma
                        liposarcoma
                        malignant granular cell myoblastoma
                        mesenchymoma
                        myoblastoma
                        myxosarcoma
                        rhabdomyosarcoma
1739   Malignant neoplasm of skin other than melanoma
        17390x Basal cell carcinoma

1739	17390x	*continued*
		Basal cell epithelioma
		Rodent ulcer
		excludes: basal cell nevus syndrome
	17391x	Adenoid squamous cell carcinoma
		Squamous cell carcinoma
		Squamous cell epithelioma
	17392x	Tar epithelioma
	17393x	Marjolin's ulcer
	17394x	Basisquamous cell carcinoma
		Basisquamous cell epithelioma
		Pseudoglandular carcinoma
	17395x	Basal cell nevus syndrome
		Gorlin's syndrome
	17396x	Malignant adnexal tumours
		includes: apocrine sweat gland carcinoma
		eccrine gland carcinoma
		sweat gland carcinoma
		sebaceous gland carcinoma
	17399x	Carcinoma of skin NOS
		Epithelioma of skin NOS
174		Malignant neoplasm of breast
	174x0x	Paget's disease of breast
		Paget's disease of nipple
	174x1x	Carcinoma of breast
2028		Other neoplasms of lymphoid tissue
	20280x	Lymphoma of skin
2088		Leukemia of unspecified cell type
	20880x	Leukemia cutis
2113		Benign neoplasm of colon
	21130x	Peutz Jeghers syndrome
	21131x	Polyposis coli
	21132x	Gardner's syndrome
	21133x	Cronkhite Canada syndrome
213		Benign neoplasm of bone and cartilage
	213x0x	Subungual exostosis
	213x1x	Chondroma
		Osteochondroma
214		Lipoma
	214x0x	Angiolipoma
		Fibrolipoma
		Lipoma NOS
	214x1x	Hibernoma
2159		Benign neoplasm of muscular and connective tissue
	21590x	Periungual fibroma
		Ungal fibroma
	21591x	Myxoma
		Synovioma
	21592x	Granular cell myoblastoma

21593x Rhabdomyoma
21594x Fibroepithelial polyp of Pinkus
21595x Fibrous papule of nose
21596x Juvenile digital fibromatosis
21597x Leiomyoma multiple
21598x Leiomyoma single
216x0 Benign neoplasm of epidermis
    216x00 Keratosis seborrheic
            Seborrheic keratosis
            Seborrheic wart
    216x01 Clear cell acanthoma of Degos
            Pale cell acanthoma of Degos
    216x02 Murrary Williams wart
    216x03 Warty dyskeratoma
    216x04 Keratoacanthoma
216x1 Benign neoplasm of hair follicles and sebaceous glands
    216x10 Brooke's disease
            Epithelioma adenoides cysticum
            Trichoepithelioma
            Trichofolliculoma
    216x11 Benign calcifying epithelioma of Malherbe
            Pilomatrixoma
    216x12 Sebaceous adenoma
            Sebaceous epithelioma
            Senile sebaceous adenoma
            Senile sebaceous hyperplasia
216x2 Benign neoplasm of sweat glands and sweat ducts
    216x20 Syringoma
    216x21 Benign cylindroma
            Turban tumor
    216x22 Other specified tumours of eccrine sweat glands
            includes: clear cell hidradenoma
                    eccrine nevus
                    eccrine poroma
                    eccrine spiradenoma
                    eruptive hidradenoma
    216x23 Other specified tumors of apocrine sweat glands
            includes: apocrine hidrocystoma
                    apocrine nevus
                    hidradenoma papilliferum
                    syringocystadenoma papilliferum
    216x24 Myoepithelioma
    216x29 Adnexal tumor NOS
216x3 Pigmented nevus
    216x30 Blue nevus
    216x31 Becker's nevus
            Pigmented hairy nevus
    216x32 Mongolian spot
    216x33 Giant pigmented nevus
            Bathing trunk nevus

216x34 Oculocutaneous nevus
      includes: Ito nevus
              Ota nevus
216x35 Juvenile melanoma
216x36 Amelanotic nevus
216x37 Cellular nevus
      includes: balloon cell nevus
              benign melanoma
              compound nevus
              junctional nevus
              pigmented nevus NOS

216x4 Other nevi of skin
216x40 Epidermal nevus
      includes: linear nevus
              nevus unius lateris
              verrucous nevus
      excludes: nevus sebaceus of Jadassohn (*see* 216x43)
216x41 Connective tissue nevus
      includes: collagenous plaques
              nevus elasticus
      excludes: juvenile elastoma (*see* 757335)
216x42 Nevus lipomatodes superficialis
      Nevus lipomatosus
      excludes: lipoma (*see* 214x0x)
216x43 Nevus sebaceus of Jadassohn

216x5 Other specified benign neoplasms of skin
216x50 Dermatofibroma
      Histiocytoma
      Sclerosing hemangioma
216x51 Dermoid cyst of skin
216x52 Fibroma of skin
216x53 Cutaneous meningioma

228 Hemangioma and lymphangioma
228x0x Port wine nevus
228x1x Glomangioma
      Glomus tumour
228x2x Benign angioendothelioma
      Benign endothelioma
      Benign hemangioendothelioma
228x3x Blue rubber bleb nevus
228x9x Angioma NOS
      Hemangioma NOS

2299 Benign neoplasm of other organs and tissues
22990x Papilloma of skin
22991x Hamartoma of skin NOS
22992x Lymphadenosis benigna cutis
      Lymphocytoma
22993x Juvenile xanthogranuloma
      Nevoxanthoendothelioma

22994x Atypical fibroxanthoma
        Reticulohistiocytoma

III Endocrine, Nutritional, Metabolic and Immunity Disorders

2468   Other disorders of thyroid
        24680x Pretibial myxedema
                Skin manifestation of hyperthyroidism
                Thyroid acropachy
2507   Diabetes mellitus with other specified manifestations
        25070x Diabetic pruritus
        25071x Necrobiosis lipoidica diabeticorum
        25072x Diabetic lipodystrophy
        25073x Diabetic xanthomatosis
                Xanthoma diabeticorum
2580   Polyglandular dysfunction and related disorders
        25800x Acrogeria
        25801x Cockayne syndrome (dwarfism)
        25802x Werner's syndrome
2702   Other disturbances of aromatic amino-acid metabolism
        27020x Albinism
        27021x Albinoidism
                Piebaldism
                Waardenburg's syndrome
                White forelock disease
        27022x Chediak Higashi disease
        27023x Alkaptonuria
2721   Other and unspecified hyperlipoproteinemia
        27210x Xanthelasma
        27211x Systemic xanthomatosis
        27212x Eruptive xanthoma
        27219x Xanthoma NOS
2727   Generalised lipoidoses
        27270x Angiokeratoma diffusum corporis
                Fabry's angiokeratoma
                Fabry's disease
        27271x Gaucher's disease
        27272x Niemann Pick disease
2728   Disorders of lipid metabolism
        27280x Lipoid dermato-arthritis
        27281x Subcutaneous fat necrosis
                excludes: neonatal fat necrosis (7781)
        27282x Hyalinosis cutis et mucosae
                Lipoid proteinosis
                Urbach's lipoid proteinosis
2771   Disorders of porphyrin metabolism
        27710x Congenital erythropoietic porphyria

73

27711x Porphyria cutanea tarda
27712x Variegate porphyria
27713x Erythropoietic protoporphyria
27714x Acquired porphyria
Secondary porphyria
Toxic porphyria
27719x Hereditary porphyria NOS
2773 Amyloidosis
27730x Amyloidosis
27731x Amyloid degeneration
27732x Lichen amyloidosus
2775 Mucopolysaccharidoses
27750x Gargoylism
Hurler syndrome
27751x Hunter syndrome
27752x Morquio disease
Morquio Brailsford syndrome
27753x Sanfilippo syndrome
27754x Scheie syndrome

IV   Diseases of the Blood and Blood-forming Organs

2866 Defibrination syndrome
28660x Purpura fulminans
2872 Other non-thrombocytopenic purpuras
28720x Pigmented purpura
Stasis purpura
28721x Traumatic purpura
includes: black heel
hemorrhage into skin
talon noir
28722x Rheumatic purpura
Toxic purpura
28723x Autoerythrocyte sensitisation
Painful bruising syndrome
Psychogenic purpura
28724x Toxic capillaritis due to drug
includes: carbromal eruption
28725x Senile and steroid purpura
2874 Secondary thrombocytopenia
28740x Kasabach Merritt syndrome
2880 Agranulocytosis
28800x Cyclic neutropenia

V   Mental Disorders

3001 Hysteria
30010x Compensation neurosis

30011x Conversion anesthesia
       Hysterical anesthesia
3002   Phobic states
       30020x Acaraphobia
              Insectophobia
              Parasitophobia
       30021x Syphilophobia

VI   Diseases of the Nervous System and Sense Organs

3518   Other facial nerve disorders
       35180x Melkersson Rosenthal syndrome
3632   Other and unspecified forms of chorioretinitis
       36320x Oculocutaneous syndrome
       36321x Vogt Koyanagi syndrome
3800   Perichondritis of pinna
       38000x Chondrodermatitis nodularis helicis

VII   Diseases of the Circulatory System

4438   Other peripheral vascular disease
       44380x Acrocyanosis
       44381x Erythromelalgia
       44382x Diabetic dermopathy
              Diabetic peripheral microangiopathy
       44383x Hypertensive ulcer
4460   Polyarteritis nodosa
       44600x Periarteritis nodosa
              Polyarteritis nodosa
       44601x Necrotising arteritis
              Necrotising vasculitis
4478   Other diseases of arteries and arterioles
       44780x Allergic vasculitis
              includes: allergic arteritis
                 angiodermatitis
                 cutaneous vasculitis
                 Gougerot trisymptome
                 hypersensitivity angiitis of skin
                 leukocytoclastic angiitis
                 leukocytoclastic vasculitis
                 nodular dermal allergide
                 purpuric vasculitis
       44781x Angiitis NEC
              excludes: disseminated vasculitis
                 infective endarteritis
                 obliterative vascular disease
       44782x Atrophie blanche

44783x Degos disease
        Malignant atrophic papulosis
4481   Non-neoplastic capillary nevus
44810x Spider nevus
       includes: nevus araneus
             spider angioma
             spider telangiectasis
44811x Campbell de Morgan spot
44812x Strawberry angioma
        Strawberry mark
        Strawberry nevus
4489   Other diseases of capillaries
44890x Telangiectasia NEC and NOS
       includes: arborising
             essential
             generalised
             primary
44891x Cutaneous capillaritis not due to a drug (*see* 28734x)
44892x Angioma NEC
       includes: vascular nevus NEC
       excludes: angioma NOS (*see* 228x9x)

IX   Diseases of the Digestive System

5285   Diseases of the lips
52850x Angular cheilitis
52851x Glandular cheilitis
52852x Cheilitis NOS
52853x Acquired hypertrophy of lip
52854x Mucous cyst of lip
52855x Blood cyst of lip

X   Disease of the Genito-Urinary System

6078   Other diseases of penis
60780x Balanitis xerotica obliterans
60781x Aphthous ulcer of penis
60782x Peyronie's disease
       includes: nonvenereal chordee
             penile plastic induration
60783x Balanitis erosiva circinata et gangrenosa (*see* 0993)
60784x Zoon's balanitis
60789x Balanitis NOS
       includes: balanoposthitis
             phagadenic balanitis
6240   Dystrophy of vulva
62400x Kraurosis of vulva
62401x Leukoplakia of vulva

Disease of the Skin and Subcutaneous Tissue

6810   Cellulitis of finger and toe
        68100x Acute paronychia
                Whitlow
                excludes: melanotic whitlow (see *172*)
        68101x Chronic paronychia
        68102x Onychia
6860   Pyoderma
        68600x Pyoderma gangrenosum
        68601x Ecthyma gangrenosum
                Meleney's ulcer
                Pyoderma vegetans
        68602x Chancriform pyoderma
                Granuloma faciale
        68603x Dermatitis gangrenosa infantum
        68609x Pyoderma NOS
6868   Other local "infections" of skin and subcutaneous tissue
        68680x Acrodermatitis atrophicans chronica
                Acrodermatitis continua
                Acrodermatitis perstans
                Acrodermatitis pustula continua (Hallopeau)
                Acropustulosis
                Dermatitis perstans
                Dermatitis repens
                Dermatitis vegetans
        68681x Acrodermatitis enteropathica
        68682x Ecthyma
                Omphalitis
                Perleche
                Sloughing skin
        68689x Fistula NOS
                Sinus NOS
                excludes: candidal infection (*see* 1120)
6918   Other infantile conditions
        69180x Atopic dermatitis
                includes: atopic eczema
                    Besnier's prurigo
                    Brocq's disease
                    diffuse neurodermatitis
                    infantile eczema
                excludes: cradle cap (*see* 69181x)
                    milk crust (*see* 69181x)
        69181x Cradle cap
                Milk crust
6923   Contact dermatitis due to a drug
        69230x Allergic contact dermatitis
        69231x Irritant contact dermatitis

69232x Drug induced photodermatitis
        Drug induced photosensitivity
69239x Contact dermatitis, type unspecified
6924   Contact dermatitis due to other chemical products
69240x Allergic contact dermatitis
69241x Irritant contact dermatitis
69242x Induced photodermatitis
        Induced photosensitivity
69249x Contact dermatitis, type unspecified
6926   Contact dermatitis due to plants
69260x Allergic contact dermatitis
        includes: poison ivy dermatitis
            primula dermatitis
            ragweed dermatitis
            rhus dermatitis
69261x Irritant contact dermatitis
69262x Phytophotodermatitis
69269x Plant dermatitis, type unspecified
6927   Dermatitis due to solar radiation
69270x Erythema ab igne
69271x Actinic cheilitis
        Actinic dermatitis
        Photodermatitis excluding that due to drug or plant
        Photosensitivity excluding that due to drug or plant
        Solar eczema
        Solar erythema
        Solar urticaria
69272x Actinic reticuloid
69273x Jessner's lymphocytic infiltration
69274x Polymorphous light eruption
69275x Sunburn
6928   Contact dermatitis due to other specified agents
69280x Allergic contact dermatitis
69281x Irritant contact dermatitis
69282x Radiodermatitis
69289x Contact dermatitis, type unspecified
6929   Other types of eczema
69290x Discoid dermatitis
        Discoid eczema
        Nummular eczema
69291x Secondary eczema
        Sensitisation dermatitis
69292x Bacterial intertrigo
        Eczematous intertrigo
69293x Eczematide
        Seborrhoeide
69294x Hand eczema NOS
        excludes: contact dermatitis (*see* 6923-6928)
            pompholyx (*see* 70580x)

78

69295x Chronic superficial dermatitis
69296x Senile dermatitis
69297x Brocq's erythrose peribuccale pigmentaire
69298x Exfoliative dermatitis
Exfoliative eczema
69299x Dermatitis NOS
Eczema NOS
6944 Pemphigus (excluding Hailey Hailey pemphigus *see* 757321)
69440x Pemphigus erythematosus
Pemphigus foliaceus
Pemphigus Senear Usher
69441x Pemphigus vulgaris
69442x Pemphigus vegetans
69443x Brazilian pemphigus
Fogo selvagem
6950 Toxic erythema
69500x Toxic eruption
Toxic erythema
excludes: toxic erythema neonatorum (7788)
69501x Fixed drug eruption
69502x Erythema annulare (Darier)
Erythema figuratum perstans
Erythema marginatum rheumaticum
69503x Palmar erythema
69504x Erythema chronicum migrans
69505x Ashy dermatosis
69506x Erythema dyschromicum perstans
Erythema gyratum perstans
Erythema gyratum repens
69507x Lichenoid drug eruption
69509x Drug eruption NOS
6951 Erythema multiforme
69510x Erythema multiforme
69511x Lyell's disease
Toxic epidermal necrolysis
69512x Ectodermosis erosiva pluriorificialis
Stevens Johnson syndrome
69513x Acute neutrophilic dermatosis
Sweet's syndrome
6952 Erythema nodosum
69520x Erythema nodosum
excludes: sarcoid as cause (see 135x2x)
tuberculosis as cause (see 01710x)
69521x Erythema induratum (Whitfield)
excludes: tuberculosis as cause (see 01711x)
6953 Rosacea
69530x Rosacea
69531x Rosaceous conjunctivitis
Rosaceous keratitis

69532x Rhinophyma
69533x Perioral dermatitis
69534x Haber's syndrome
6958 Other specified erythematous conditions
69580x Erythema elevatum diutinum
Extracellular cholesterolosis
69581x Granuloma annulare
69582x Granuloma multiforme (Leiker)
69583x Lipomelanic reticulosis
69584x Exfoliation
6961 Psoriasis
69610x Psoriasis
Psoriatic intertrigo
69611x Pustular psoriasis of palms and soles
69612x Generalised pustular psoriasis
6962 Parapsoriasis
69620x Parapsoriasis en gouttes
Parapsoriasis guttate
Pityriasis lichenoides chronica
69621x Mucha Habermann disease
Pityriasis lichenoides varioliformis et acuta
69622x Parapsoriasis variegata
Parakeratosis variegata
69623x Parapsoriasis en plaques
6963 Pityriasis rosea
69630x Pityriasis rosea
69631x Pityriasis circinata
Pityriasis rotunda
6969 Other types of pityriasis
69690x Acroerythème pustuleux
Gianotti Crosti syndrome
Papular eruption of childhood
6983 Lichenification
69830x Lichen simplex
Lichenification
69831x Pseudoepitheliomatous hyperplasia
69832x Prurigo nodularis
6984 Dermatitis factitia
69840x Artefact
Dermatitis artefacta
Self-mutilation
69841x Neurotic excoriations
6988 Other pruritic conditions
69880x Senile pruritus
69881x Winter itch
69882x Generalised pruritus
7010 Circumscribed scleroderma
70100x Lichen sclerosus et atrophicus

70101x Localised scleroderma
        Morphea
70102x Pasini et Pierini atrophoderma
7011   Acquired keratoderma
70110x Acquired ichthyosis
        Acquired xeroderma
70111x Keratoderma climactericum
70112x Keratosis blenorrhagica (see 0993)
70113x Keratosis punctata
70114x Stucco keratosis
        Tar keratosis
70115x Hyperkeratosis follicularis in cutem penetrans
        Kyrle's disease
70116x Elastosis perforans serpiginosa
        Miescher's elastoma
70117x Arsenical wart
7013   Striae atrophicae
70130x Striae albicantes
        Striae atrophicae
        Striae distensae
70131x Anetoderma
        includes: atrophic spots
                focal dermal hypoplasia
                follicular atrophoderma
                macular atrophy
                Schweninger Buzzi anetoderma
70132x Striae due to corticosteroid therapy
7018   Other hypertrophic and atrophic conditions of skin
70180x Actinic elastosis
        includes: cutis rhomboidalis nuchae
                elastosis
                senile skin
                solar elastosis
70181x Acquired dermatolysis
        includes: acquired dermatorrhexis
                acquired elastic skin
                dermatitis atrophicans diffusa
70182x Nodular elastosis with cysts and comedones
70183x Atrophoderma vermiculata
        includes: folliculitis erythematosa reticulata
70184x Ulerythema ophryogenes
70185x Arndt Gottron syndrome
        includes: focal mucinosis
                lichen myxedematosus
                papular mucinosis
                scleromyxedema
70186x Acrochordon
        includes: acquired skin tags

70187x Pachyderma
    includes: pachydermoperiostosis
70188x Confluent and reticulate papillomatosis
702 Other dermatoses
702x0x Cornu cutaneum
    Cutaneous horn
702x1x Hutchinson's lentigo
    includes: Hutchinson's melanosis
        Dubreuilh's melanosis circumscripta
        lentigo maligna
702x2x Leukokeratosis of lip (vermilion portion)
    includes: smoker's lip
702x3x Senile keratosis
    Solar keratosis
702x9x Precancerous dermatosis NOS or NEC
7038 Other diseases of nail
70380x Nail biting
70381x Koilonychia
    includes: spoon nail
70382x Beau's lines
70383x Splinter hemorrhage
70384x Onycholysis
70385x Onychogryphosis
70386x Yellow nail syndrome
70387x Pitting of nails
70388x Other specified nail dystrophies
    includes: acquired anonychia
        acquired brittle nails
        acquired nail dystrophy
        acquired onychodystrophy
        atrophy of nails
        defluvium unguium
        discoloration of nail
        egg shell nails
        fragilitas unguium
        leukopathia unguium
        lamellar onycholysis
        pterygium of nail
        shedding of nails
        splitting of nails
70389x Nail dystrophy NOS
70400 Alopecia due to physical agent
704000 Trichotillomania
704001 Traction alopecia
    includes: traumatic alopecia (physical)
    excludes: trichotillomania (see 704000)
704002 Chemical alopecia
    includes: traumatic alopecia (chemical)
    excludes: alopecia due to drugs (see 704003)

82

	704003	Alopecia due to drugs
	704004	Alopecia due to radiotherapy
70401		Alopecia due to other causes
	704010	Biological alopecia

704003 Alopecia due to drugs
704004 Alopecia due to radiotherapy
70401 Alopecia due to other causes
   704010 Biological alopecia
      includes: androgenetic alopecia
          constitutional alopecia
          female alopecia
          male alopecia
   704011 Telogen effluvium
      includes: postinflammatory alopecia
          postpartum alopecia
   704012 Alopecia areata
      includes: alopecia totalis
          alopecia universalis
   704013 Cicatricial alopecia
      includes: pseudopelade
   704014 Alopecia mucinosa
      includes: follicular mucinosis
   704015 Acquired hypotrichosis
   704016 Aminogenic alopecia
7048 Other diseases of hair and hair follicles
   70480x Irritant folliculitis
   70481x Ingrowing hair
         Pili incarnati
   70482x Folliculitis decalvans
      includes: perifolliculitis capitis abscedens
   70489x Hair anomaly NOS or NEC
7058 Other disorders of sweat glands
   70580x Cheiropompholyx
      includes: dyshidrotic eczema
          pompholyx
   70581x Hidradenitis suppurativa
   70582x Bromhidrosis
         Chromidrosis
         Osmidrosis
   70583x Apocrine acne
         Fox Fordyce disease
   70584x Granulosa rubra nasi
7061 Other acne
   70610x Acne vulgaris
      includes: blackhead
         comedo
         cystic acne
   70611x Acne infantum
         Infantile acne
   70612x Chloracne
         Oil acne
         Tar acne

70613x Acne indurata
          includes: acne keloid
                    dermatitis papillaris capillitii
70614x Tropical acne
70615x Acne agminata
70616x Acne excoriée des jeunes filles
70617x Acne vulgaris due to corticosteroid therapy
70618x Halogen eruption
          includes: bromacne
                    iododerma
7062   Sebaceous cyst
70620x Epidermal cyst
          includes: implantation cyst
                    inclusion cyst
                    milium
                    pilar cyst
                    sebaceous cyst
                    wen
                    whitehead
70621x Sebocystomatosis
          Steatocystoma multiplex
7078   Chronic ulcer of other unspecified sites
70780x Neuropathic ulcer
          includes: perforating ulcer
                    trophic ulcer
70781x Desert sore
          includes: veldt sore
70782x Tropical ulcer
7083   Dermatographic urticaria
70830x Dermographism
70831x Pressure urticaria
7088   Other specified urticaria
70880x Chronic urticaria
70881x Acute urticaria NOS
70882x Aquagenic urticaria
70900   Dyschromia, increased pigmentation
709000 Benign lentigo
          includes: ephelides
                    freckle
709001 Café au lait spot
709002 Melanosis:
          includes: chloasma
                    melanoderma
                    melasma
                    senile melanosis
709003 Racial pigmentation – symptomatic
709004 Toxic melanosis
          includes: melanodermatitis toxica

84

continued

709004   Riehl's melanosis
               tar melanosis
709005 Poikiloderma of Civatte
709006 Tattoo
709007 Occupational melanosis
             Occupational pigmentation
709008 Dyschromia due to metal
         includes: arsenical pigmentation
               hyperpigmentation due to metal
               hypopigmentation due to metal
709009 Pigmentation NOS

70901   Dyschromia, decreased pigmentation
709010 Vitiligo
         includes: Alezzandrini's syndrome
709011 Nevus anemicus
         includes: acromia cutis
709012 Sutton's nevus
         includes: halo nevus
               leukoderma acquisitum centrifugum
709013 Postinflammatory pigmentation
         includes: hyperpigmentation
               hypopigmentation

7091   Vascular disorders
70910x Angioma serpiginosum
70911x Bloom's syndrome
             Poikiloderma of Bloom
70912x Pigmented purpuric eruptions
         includes: Gougerot Blum syndrome

               lichen aureus
               lichenoid purpuric pigmented dermatitis
               Majocchi's disease
               purpura annularis telangiectoides
               Schamberg's disease
70913x Poikiloderma atrophicans vasculare (Jacobi)

7093   Degenerative skin disorders
70930x Cutaneous calcification
         includes: calcinosis circumscripta
               calcinosis cutis
               calcinosis universalis
               dystrophic calcification
               osteoma cutis
               pinnal calcification
70931x Colloid milium
70932x Colloid degeneration of skin

7098   Other diseases of the skin
70980x Dermatosis papulosa nigra
70981x Chafing
         includes: chapping

7098   *continued*
　　　　70981x   lip sucking
　　　　　　　　 thumb sucking
　　　　70982x   Occupational stigma
　　　　70983x   Hutchinson's spring eruption
　　　　　　　　 includes: hydroa aestivale
　　　　　　　　　　 hydroa vacciniforme
　　　　　　　　　　 juvenile spring eruption
　　　　　　　　　　 prurigo aestivale
　　　　　　　　　　 spring eruption
　　　　70984x   Necrobiosis lipoidica (not associated with diabetes)
　　　　　　　　 includes: granuloma disciformis
　　　　70985x   Granulomatous necrosis
　　　　70986x   Staphylococcal granuloma
　　　　70987x   Eosinophilic cellulitis
　　　　70988x   Foreign body granuloma
　　　　　　　　 includes: beryllium granuloma
　　　　　　　　　　 ear piercing granuloma
　　　　　　　　　　 friction granuloma
　　　　　　　　　　 lipophagic granuloma
　　　　　　　　　　 oil granuloma
　　　　　　　　　　 paraffinoma
　　　　　　　　　　 sea urchin granuloma
　　　　　　　　　　 talc granuloma
　　　　　　　　　　 zirconium granuloma

XIII   Diseases of the Musculoskeletal System and Connective Tissue

7108   Other diffuse diseases of connective tissue
　　　　71080x   Scleredema
　　　　　　　　 includes: Buschke's scleredema

XIV   Congenital Anomalies

7428   Specified congenital anomalies of nervous system
　　　　74280x   Melanocytosis
　　　　　　　　 includes: intracranial melanocytosis
　　　　　　　　　　 meningeal melanocytosis
　　　　　　　　　　 neurocutaneous melanosis
　　　　　　　　　　 Riley Day syndrome
7438   Congenital anomalies of eye
　　　　74380x   heterochromia
　　　　74381x   Excess skin of eyelid
　　　　74382x   Dyschromatosis symmetrical
　　　　　　　　 Dyschromatosis universalis

7508	Congenital anomalies of upper alimentary tract

7508   Congenital anomalies of upper alimentary tract
          75080x Fordyce condition (of mouth and lips)
                  excludes: aberrant sebaceous glands on genitalia
          75081x Oral epithelial nevus
                  White sponge nevus

7528   Congenital anomalies of genital organs
          75280x Hirsuties papillaris penis
                  Pearly penile papules
          75281x Fordyce condition (of genitalia)
                  excludes: aberrant sebaceous glands of mouth and lips

7556   Congenital anomalies of limbs
          75560x Nail patella syndrome
                  includes: absent patella
                  patella nail syndrome

7564   Congenital anomalies of musculoskeletal system
          75640x Maffucci's syndrome
                  includes: dyschondroplasia with hemangiomata

7568   Other specified anomalies of muscle, tendon, fascia and connective
                  tissue
          75680x Ehlers Danlos syndrome
                  includes: chalazoderma
                  congenital dermatolysis
                  congenital dermatorrhexis
                  congenital lax skin

7571   Ichthyosis
          75710x Ichthyosis vulgaris (dominant inheritance)
          75711x Ichthyosis vulgaris (sex-linked recessive inheritance)
          75712x Other specified forms of ichthyosis
                  includes: alligator skin disease
                  harlequin fetus
                  ichthyosiform erythroderma:
                    bullous type
                    nonbullous type
                    Sjögren Larsen
                  ichthyosis congenita
                  ichthyosis fetalis
                  ichthyosis follicularis
                  ichthyosis hystrix
                  keratosis exfoliativa
                  lamellar ichthyosis
          75713x Netherton syndrome
          75714x Rud syndrome
          75715x Tylosis
                  includes: keratosis circumscripta
                  Keratosis palmaris et plantaris
                  Mal de Meleda
                  Mljet disease
                  Papillon Lefevre

7571 *continued*
  75713x polykeratosis of Touraine
      Thost Unna syndrome
  75719x Ichthyosis NOS
75730 Specified anomalies of skin
  757300 Pseudoxanthoma elasticum
  757301 Benign acanthosis nigricans
      includes: congenital acanthosis nigricans
      excludes: acquired acanthosis nigricans (see 7012)
        pseudoacanthosis nigricans (see 757302)
  757302 Pseudoacanthosis nigricans
75731 Dyskeratotic conditions
  757310 Dyskeratosis congenita
  757311 Darier's disease
      Keratosis follicularis
  757312 Keratosis pilaris
  757313 Angiokeratoma of Fordyce
      Angiokeratoma of Mibelli
  757314 Congenital xeroderma
  757315 Porokeratosis of Mibelli
  757316 Erythrokeratoderma variabilis
  757317 Acrokeratosis verruciformis
      includes: epidermodysplasia verruciformis
  757318 Comedo nevus
      Nevus comedonicus
  757319 Lichen spinulosus
75732 Bullous diseases
  757320 Epidermolysis bullosa
      includes: Cockayne syndrome
        dystrophic epidermolysis bullosa
        lethal epidermolysis bullosa
        simple epidermolysis bullosa
  757321 Chronic benign familial pemphigus
      Hailey Hailey disease
  757322 Bloch Sulzberger disease
      Incontinentia pigmenti
75733 Other specified disease of skin
  757330 Xeroderma pigmentosum
      includes: de Sanctis Cacchione syndrome
  757331 Urticaria pigmentosa
      includes: mast cell disease
        mastocytosis
        telangiectasia macularis perstans
  757332 Thomson's disease
      includes: congenital poikiloderma
        Rothmund Thomson disease
  757333 Ectodermal dysplasia
      includes: anidrotic ectodermal dysplasia
        congenital ectodermal defect
        hidrotic ectodermal dysplasia

757334 Oral-facial-digital syndrome
757335 Juvenile elastoma
     includes: perforating elastoma
757336 Cutis verticis gyrata
     includes: gyrate scalp
757337 Aplasia of skin
     includes: agenesis of skin
          congenital absence of skin
          congenital scalp defect
757338 Congenital accessory skin tag (acquired 70186x)
7574 Specified anomalies of hair
75740x Congenital alopecia
     includes: agenesis of hair
          atrichia congenita
          Marie Unna hypotrichosis
75741x Congenital hirsuties
75742x Congenital canities
75743x Beaded hair
     includes: monilethrix
          pili annulati
          pili torti
          ringed hair
          trichostasis spinulosa
75744x Hair follicle nevus
     Woolly hair nevus
75745x Congenital dystrophies
     includes: allotrichia circumscriptum
          bamboo hair
          fragilitas crinum
          trichonodosis
          trichorrhexis nodosa
75749x Hair anomaly NOS
7575 Specified anomalies of nail
75750x Pachyonychia congenita
75751x Agenesis of nail
     includes: congenital anonychia
          Congenital atrophy of nail
75752x Congenital onychodystrophy
     includes: brittle nails
          furrowing of nails
          koilonychia
75759x Congenital anomaly of nail NOS
7596 Other hamartoses NEC
75960x Arteriovenous angiomatosis
     excludes: arteriovenous aneurysm (see 7476)
75961x Sturge Weber syndrome
     includes: encephalocutaneous angiomatosis
          encephalofacial angiomatosis
75962x Klippel Trenaunay Weber syndrome

7598   Other specified syndrome
        75980x   Marfan's syndrome
                 includes: arachnodactyly
        75981x   Oculoauricular vertebral dysplasia
        75982x   Oculolentodigital dysplasia
        75983x   Bonnet Dechaume Blanc syndrome
        75984x   Lentiginoses syndrome
        75989x   Other specified syndromes NEC

XVII   Injury and Poisoning

9990   Vaccination of smallpox, complications
        99900x   Accidental vaccination
        99901x   Eczema vaccinatum
                 includes: Kaposi's varicelliform eruption
        99902x   Generalised vaccinia
        99903x   Vaccinia gangrenosa
        99904x   Complication of vaccination NEC
        99909x   Complication of vaccination NOS
9993   Complication of other inoculated infection
        99930x   BCG granuloma
9994   Allergic reactions to therapy
        99940x   Anaphylactic reaction to serum
        99941x   Herxheimer reaction
        99942x   Arthus phenomenon
        99943x   Shwartzmann reaction

International Coding Index for Dermatology